Toward a Healthier Garden State

Toward a Healthier Garden State

Beyond Cancer Clusters and COVID

MICHAEL R. GREENBERG AND
DONA SCHNEIDER

Rutgers University Press

New Brunswick, Camden, and Newark, New Jersey

London and Oxford

Rutgers University Press is a department of Rutgers, The State University of New Jersey, one of the leading public research universities in the nation. By publishing worldwide, it furthers the University's mission of dedication to excellence in teaching, scholarship, research, and clinical care.

Library of Congress Cataloging-in-Publication Data

Names: Greenberg, Michael R., author. | Schneider, Dona, 1946– author.
Title: Toward a healthier Garden State : beyond cancer clusters and COVID / Michael R. Greenberg and Dona Schneider.
Description: New Brunswick : Rutgers University Press, [2023] | Includes bibliographical references and index.
Identifiers: LCCN 2022035163 | ISBN 9781978832008 (paperback) | ISBN 9781978832015 (hardback) | ISBN 9781978832022 (epub) | ISBN 9781978832046 (pdf)
Subjects: LCSH: Public health—New Jersey. | Health planning—New Jersey.
Classification: LCC RA447.N57 G74 2023 | DDC 362.109749—dc23/eng/20221122
LC record available at https://lccn.loc.gov/2022035163

A British Cataloging-in-Publication record for this book is available from the British Library.

♾ The paper used in this publication meets the requirements of the American National Standard for Information Sciences—Permanence of Paper for Printed Library Materials, ANSI Z39.48-1992.

rutgersuniversitypress.org

Contents

Preface

We had two reasons for writing a book about upstream factors and public health in New Jersey. First, New Jersey's healthcare sector is massive; the state added almost a quarter-million new jobs in health care since 1990. Although pharmaceuticals and life sciences are not considered part of this employment sector, they are part of New Jersey's overall health-related economy and remain the fastest growing industries in the state. Additionally, thousands of students across the state are studying public health, medicine, biomedical engineering, environmental science, and other health-related disciplines. In short, one reason for writing this book is the large audience of individuals who work in health care, pharma, life sciences, and the related areas of environmental protection, urban planning, transportation, housing, social work, and the many jobs directly and indirectly connected to the social, economic, political, and environmental determinants of health.

The second reason for writing this book is to advocate for a Health in All Policies approach to public policy.[1-6] This approach requires that public policies be evaluated for their ramifications on the health of the population, not just the health of the economy or selected groups. To build our case, we decided to begin this book by examining the forces that joined together to improve public health in New Jersey after World War II. We settled on this focus because innumerable personal, corporate, and government decisions have brought New Jersey from distressed cities and a "Cancer Alley" label to the promise of a brighter and healthier future. Baby boomers born between 1946 and 1964 may remember many of the events and policy decisions described in this book, but younger readers will have less familiarity with what happened along the way. Thus, we feel it is important to closely reflect on what worked and what may have made things worse in the public health and healthcare arenas so we can more effectively address those daunting challenges in the foreseeable future.

New Jersey's progress has been slowed and accelerated by events and policies—upstream factors that influence health but are beyond the control of individuals. We present one or more events in each chapter that were part obstacle and part opportunity. The Cancer Alley presentation in chapter 4, for example, emphasizes interdisciplinary contributions from the literature, data with some statistical massaging, and it blends interviews from officials of that period. We used this approach to flesh out the policies and other events that created and later quelled the Cancer Alley moniker for New Jersey. Chapter 5 zeroes in on COVID-19's hellacious impacts, especially on poor minorities living in the state's older cities, and the efforts to respond. Chapter 6 illustrates the role of policy-makers and the New Jersey Supreme Court, specifically how their interventions attempted to provide more educational and housing opportunities for residents with limited means.

Throughout the book we specifically point out instances where adverse public health consequences could have been avoided or significantly reduced if health had been a more serious consideration in the decision-making process. These instances are the inflection points that make our case for Health in All Policies and the importance of building a "culture of health" that supports this important concept. We also wrestled with how much attention should be paid to long-standing risks, including corruption, social inequality, and blind adherence to populism—issues that have been with us for centuries.

Although this book does not focus on long-standing risks, it also does not ignore them, particularly because issues with income, education, housing, and access to health care have long been present even as new challenges such as unprecedented addiction levels, climate change, cyber risks, financial failures, and disease pandemics have emerged. Therefore, every chapter looks for evidence of long-standing and emerging risks, and we place special emphasis in the epilogue on the ones we are likely to face going forward.

We acknowledge that health is substantially influenced by age, gender, genetics, and other personal attributes, as well as by individual lifestyle decisions and social and community networks. We do not ignore these personal health determinants, but they are not the focus of this book. Instead, we focus on the broader set of upstream factors defined as policies and actions influencing design, land use, transportation, energy, housing, infrastructure, decisions by government officials at all levels, businesses, and, more recently, decisions by not-for-profit organizations. Such decisions have consequences that impact the health of us all as well as that of select (particularly high-risk) individuals.

We also acknowledge that while the Garden State has been the scene of some terrible health-related events, it has also come up with some of the best solutions to public health challenges and important innovations. For example, the concrete barriers developed for traffic safety along Route 1 (called Jersey barriers) are now deployed across the globe for highway safety. Similarly, during the Cancer Alley decade, state officials created the New Jersey Carcinogen Survey, a data set of potential toxic exposures that served as a model for the U.S. Environmental Protection Agency's Toxic Release Inventory (TRI). Today, individuals can search that data set for hazardous industrial emissions by geographic area.[7]

At the time of this writing, the COVID-19 pandemic has shifted to endemic status—the state has been learning from this experience, but we have more to learn. The nation must engage in the struggle to retain what we have learned from this experience before the next challenge that surely will follow emerges. Alas, the reality that New Jersey cumulatively has had some of the worst outcomes from COVID-19 has stimulated considerable thinking, research, and policy development and implementation. As in many other instances, the state was hit as hard or harder than other places at the beginning of the epidemic and responded aggressively. Other populations, as well as our own, will benefit from our travail. In other words, there are many lessons to be learned from New Jersey's public health legacy as well as its healthier future.

Readers of this book should come away with (1) the recent public health history of the most densely developed, and one of the most affluent and demographically diverse states in the nation; and (2) the importance of managing upstream social, political, economic, and environmental factors to improve the public's health. Notably, they should understand the importance of Health in All Policies and developing a culture of health to aggressively and fearlessly push down the road toward a healthier New Jersey.

MRG, DS
August 23, 2022

References

1 World Health Organization (WHO). The 8th Global Conference on Health Promotion, Helsinki, Finland, 10–14 June 2013. Updated April 23, 2014. https://www.who.int/teams/health-promotion/enhanced-wellbeing/eighth-global-conference

2 Association of State and Territorial Health Officials (ASTHO). Health in All Policies: State Public Health. Updated 2022. Accessed September 21, 2021. https://www.astho.org/HiAP/

3 Centers for Disease Control and Prevention. Health in All Policies. Updated June 9, 2016. Accessed September 21, 2021. https://www.cdc.gov/policy/hiap/index.html

4 National Association of County and City Health Officials (NACCHO). Health in All Policies. Updated 2021. Accessed September 21, 2021. https://www.naccho.org/programs/community-health/healthy-community-design/health-in-all-policies

5 National Environmental Health Association (NEHA). Health in All Policies. Updated 2022. Accessed September 21, 2021. https://www.neha.org/eh-topic/health-all-policies-hiap

6 World Health Organization (WHO). Health in All Policies: framework for country action. January 2014. https://www.afro.who.int/sites/default/files/2017-06/140120HPRHiAPFramework.pdf

7 Environmental Protection Agency (EPA). Toxics Release Inventory (TRI) Program: TRI data and tools. Updated August 25, 2022. Accessed September 21, 2021. https://www.epa.gov/toxics-release-inventory-tri-program/tri-data-and-tools

Toward a Healthier Garden State

1

Defining, Measuring, and Improving Health

━━━━━━━━━━━━━━━━━━━━━━━━━━━━●

Historically, definitions of health focused on outcomes that measure the absence of health in populations—typically death, disease, and injury rates. In the latter part of the twentieth century, definitions of health moved to include quality-of-life metrics. Today, definitions of health often include the capacity of institutions to manage health, including provisions for injury and disease prevention, as well as proactive measures by institutions to increase population wellness and well-being.

This chapter has six major goals:

1   Define health.
2   Review the metrics used to measure health in the United States.
3   Define behavioral, social, and upstream determinants of health and the complex causal pathways that link them with health outcomes.
4   Describe the history of growth in healthcare costs.
5   Examine the development of Health in All Policies, the culture of health philosophy, and risks that pose public health challenges.
6   Summarize each chapter of the book.

Dimensions of Health

Twenty-first century definitions used by both health professionals and the public recognize multiple dimensions of health, albeit there is no single agreed-upon list. We begin with the 1948 World Health Organization (WHO) statement that "health is a state of complete physical, mental and social well-being and not merely the absence of disease or infirmity."[1] What is important about this statement is that it included mental and social well-being for the first time. The definition of mental health includes a variety of personal assets, such as awareness of oneself and the surrounding environment, the ability to cope with stress and controlling one's emotions, and the ability to communicate verbally and through other forms of communication. Mental health also has spiritual, perception, and value elements, such as the ability express feelings, love, trust, selflessness, and a long list of other attributes that aid individuals in rebounding from distressing experiences and enjoying a good quality of life.[2-4] Social well-being involves functioning with others in multiple venues and at multiple times. It recognizes that some individuals are unable to cope with family or social gatherings, achieve a work–life balance, or feel safe and secure in their environments.

Prior to the 1948 definition, the physical dimensions of the health dominated health metrics for centuries. The simplest indicators of population health were the most widely used: death rates and life expectancy. Today we collect a great deal more health-related information, particularly at the individual level. We collect information on an individual's physical state (e.g., height, weight, blood pressure, laboratory, and radiology results), risk factors associated with morbidity and mortality (e.g., smoking, alcohol and drug abuse, physical activity, and nutrition), and on other factors that could undermine health (e.g., mental health status, access to health care).[2,3] As this chapter will show, however, most of the metrics reported on the health of the public continue to reflect the physical dimensions of health.

Although there is a large literature on the definitions of health, there has been no resolution about which definition is best. Ereshefsky,[5] a philosopher, argues that we are being diverted from consensus by focusing on absolutes. Instead, he argues, we should focus on descriptions of physiological and psychological states compared to norms. The U.S. government has moved toward setting goals and judging progress toward those goals by comparing the current health status of the population to norms established through metrics.

Measuring Health with Metrics

In July 1979, *Healthy People: The Surgeon General's Report on Health Promotion and Disease Prevention* started the process of establishing quantifiable health outcomes goals for the United States.[6] Building on an idea that originated in Canada, the 1979 U.S. report offered five objectives for improving Americans' health, denoting the importance of health promotion and disease prevention in achieving these goals. Shortly thereafter, *Promoting Health/Preventing Disease: Objectives for the Nation*[7] listed and described 226 measurable health objectives and an overall plan to reach them.

When written, the authors of the latter report knew that many of the objectives set out in the documents would not be met by the 1990 target year. Despite this, in 1987 the U.S. Public Health Service (PHS) began preparing the year 2000 health objectives for the nation. The process involved reaching out to key stakeholders, including state and private organizations and citizen groups. The Institute of Medicine and the PHS invited participation by hundreds of national organizations as well as all state and territorial health departments. Meetings, mailings, and hearings produced voluminous materials that led to twenty-one priority metric areas. The PHS redrafted objectives in each priority area with the help of subject matter experts. In turn, the redrafted objectives were reviewed.

The final product listing the year 2000 objectives for the nation involved more than 7,000 organizations and individuals, including one of the authors of this book, Michael Greenberg, who submitted testimony and also reviewed drafts.[8] The extensive participation by representatives of state and local governments, academic institutions, business and labor, and community and professional organizations implies that the federal government wanted to build a network of participants. In addition to building an interconnected group, the year 2000 report added a section on the human immunodeficiency virus (HIV), a disease that had yet to be well understood when the 1990 report was written. In other words, new knowledge led to significant updates in the year 2000 report. Yet in their final format the Healthy People 2000 objectives proposed five measurable goals that were not remarkably different from those of the Healthy People report in 1979.[6-8] These included:

- Reduce infant mortality to no more than seven deaths per 1,000 live births (baseline: 10.4 per 1,000 in 1986).
- Increase life expectancy to at least 78 years (baseline: 74.9 years in 1987).
- Reduce disability caused by chronic conditions to a prevalence of no more than 6 percent of all persons (age-adjusted baseline: 8.9 percent).
- Increase years of healthy life to at least 65 years (baseline: an estimated 60 years in 1987).
- Decrease the disparity in life expectancy between white and minority populations to no more than 4 years (baseline: 5.8 years in 1987).

The report had an increased emphasis on (1) preventing morbidity and disability; (2) targeting high-risk populations to reduce premature death, disease, and disability; and (3) suggesting more screening to facilitate early detection in order to prevent early death or disability.[9] Several national public health entities came together to aid states and local health agencies with implementing strategies to achieve the goals that meet their own local needs by publishing *Model Standards: A Guide for Community Preventive Health Services.*[10]

Other updates of Healthy People have occurred with targets for the years 2010[11] and 2020.[12] The 2020 report clearly expanded on the earlier ones, with 1,200 health objectives in forty-two topical areas. The Office of Disease Prevention and Health Promotion at the Centers for Disease Control and Prevention (CDC) recognized that the number of national health objectives listed for Healthy People 2020 had been overwhelming, so they developed a shorter list of twenty-six leading health indicators (see Table 1.1).[13] The list includes a broad set of indicators that effect physical, mental, and social health, including some listed as high priority that were unexpected.

These outcome indicators are directly and indirectly tied to upstream and social determinants of health. Specifically, upstream determinants are macroscale factors that comprise the social-structural influences on health and health systems; government policies; and the social, physical, economic and environmental factors that determine health.[14] Social determinants are

Table 1.1

Year 2020 Leading Health Indicators

1. Access to Health Services
   - Persons with medical insurance
   - Persons with a usual primary care provider

2. Clinical Preventive Services
   - Adults receiving colorectal cancer screening based on the most recent guidelines
   - Adults with hypertension whose blood pressure is under control
   - Persons with diagnosed diabetes whose A1c value is greater than 9 percent
   - Children receiving the recommended doses of DTaP, polio, MMR, Hib, HepB, varicella and PCV vaccines by age 19–35 months

3. Environmental Quality
   - Air Quality Index > 100
   - Children exposed to secondhand smoke

4. Injury and Violence
   - Injury deaths
   - Homicides

5. Maternal, Infant, and Child Health
   - All infant deaths
   - Total preterm live births

6. Mental Health
   - Suicide
   - Adolescents with a major depressive episode in the past 12 months

7. Nutrition, Physical Activity, and Obesity
   - Adults meeting aerobic physical activity and muscle-strengthening objectives
   - Obesity among adults
   - Obesity among children and adolescents
   - Mean daily intake of total vegetables

8. Oral Health
   - Children, and lessons, and adults who visited the dentist in the past year

9. Reproductive and Sexual Health
   - Sexually experienced females receiving reproductive health services
   - Knowledge of serostatus among HIV-positive persons

10. Social Determinants
    - Students graduating from high school within 4 years of starting 9th grade

11. Substance Abuse
    - Adolescents using alcohol or illicit drugs in the past 30 days
    - Binge drinking in the past month—Adults

12. Tobacco
    - Adult cigarette smoking
    - Adolescent cigarette smoking in the past 30 days

Abbreviations: DTaP, diphtheria, tetanus, and whooping cough (pertussis); HepB, hepatitis B; Hib, *Haemophilus influenzae* type b; HIV, human immunodeficiency virus; MMR, measles, mumps and rubella; PCV, pneumococcal disease. varicella, chicken pox.
SOURCE: Office of Disease Prevention and Health Promotion, U.S. Centers for Disease Control and Prevention.[13]

conditions in the places where people live, learn, work, and play that affect a wide range of health risks and outcomes.[15] Causal pathways linking these determinants with health are long and complex, often involving multiple intervening factors along the way, making them a challenge to study and ultimately address.[16]

There is no doubt that the CDC, other federal governmental organizations, state governments, and other institutions have put processes in place that aid in measuring progress toward the Healthy People objectives. The input and metrics gathered by these and other stakeholders continue to be important for the year 2030 objectives, which were launched nationally on August 18, 2020.[17] At that time, the New Jersey launch was already underway.

The 2030 Healthy People initiative sets out five overarching goals, along with the metrics for achieving them:

1 Attain healthy, thriving lives and well-being, free of preventable disease, disability, injury, and premature death.
2 Eliminate health disparities, achieve health equity, and attain health literacy to improve the health and well-being of all.
3 Create social, physical, and economic environments that promote attaining full potential for health and well-being for all.
4 Promote healthy development, healthy behaviors, and well-being across all life stages.
5 Engage leadership, key constituents, and the public across multiple sectors to take action and design policies that improve the health and well-being of all.

Evaluating Progress with Metrics

Advances in survey methods, data gathering, and cloud storage now allow researchers to access data sets that could not be readily weaved together in the past. For instance, the Global Burden of Disease (GBD) project uses multiple data sets to paint portraits of health and the factors that contribute to health.[18–23] The United States, its states, and other countries have access to relatively standardized traditional measurements of physical health: total deaths, crude death rates (total deaths divided by persons at risk), and age-adjusted death rates (deaths adjusted by the age profile of the nation as a whole).

Crude death rates for the nation have been calculated for more than a century; however, they are problematic because the U.S. population is aging, and some states have much younger populations than their counterparts. For example, Alaska has a relatively young population and thus a low crude death rate. By contrast, Florida has a relatively older population and a higher crude death rate. In order to compare death rates for these states, age adjustment is clearly necessary. Similarly, epidemiologists calculate separate death rates for men and women (gender-specific death rates) and increasingly for groups divided by standard census categories of race/ethnicity.

In addition to the traditional indicators of health measured by death, the United States and many other countries have begun to gather many other informative health indicators:

- Healthy life expectancy (HLE, or the number of years that a person can expect to live in good health, starting with the individual's current age).
- Years of potential life lost due to premature mortality (YPLL, or the years of life not achieved compared with a normative population goal).
- Disability-adjusted life years (DALYs, or the years lived without disability-adjusted to a normative population goal).
- Quality-adjusted life years (QALYs, or years lived within a good quality of life).
- Summary exposure preventive risk (a risk-weighted estimate of exposures).

Using data collected from 1990 and 2016, a systematic analysis by the U.S. Burden of Disease Collaborators paints a fascinating portrait of the puzzle that now characterizes U.S. health outcomes.[24,25] Beginning with the most basic, the U.S. age-adjusted death rate fell from 745.2 to 578 per 100,000 people between 1990 and 2016. With regard to the most frequent causes of death, the majority of the top 25 causes of death in 1990 were unchanged or only slightly changed in 2016. For example, ischemic heart diseases and trachea bronchus and lung cancer ranked 1 and 2, respectively, in both time periods. However, there were some interesting changes:

- Alzheimer's disease and other diseases of dementia rose from rank 7 to rank 4.
- Diabetes rose from rank 12 to rank 8.

- Opioid-related deaths rose from rank 52 to rank 15.
- Chronic kidney disease due to diabetes rose from rank 35 to rank 16.

For individuals living with disabilities, the pattern of health-related issues was relatively stable. For instance, low back pain and major depressive disorders ranked 1 and 2, respectively, in 1990 and again in 2016. However, diabetes mellitus increased from rank 8 to rank 3. At the global level, diabetes mellitus was chosen by Chinese experts as the number one cause of preventable diseases.[26] Obesity and lack of exercise are presumed to be the major precipitating factors for the development of diabetes, but not the only ones in the United States, the People's Republic of China, and many other places.[27-35]

State Health Rankings

Although this book focuses on health outcomes in New Jersey, we need to begin with a comparison among the states to put New Jersey's status in context. Americans focus a great deal on international comparisons because the United States spends much more than any other nation on health care. It is, however, not even near the top of nations in terms of better health outcomes. Over the last several decades, reducing health care expenses and focusing on more effective spending have been highly publicized and politicized topics. We argue that the underlying causes (upstream and social determinants) of poor health and death are even more important to focus on, particularly when comparing outcomes at the state level.[34] For example, twenty-one of the fifty American states demonstrated increased death rates in the twenty- to fifty-five-year-old age group between 1990 and 2016, a shocking change.[36] The contributing factors will not surprise those who follow the newspapers and other media, including the enormous increases in deaths due to substance abuse,[37] self-harm,[38-40] nonalcoholic fatty liver disease,[41,42] and other causes[35,43-45] that Case and Deaton labeled "deaths of despair."[36] These were predicted to rise in 2020 and 2021 due to the mental health crisis exacerbated by the COVID-19 pandemic.[46]

U.S. News & World Report ranks states in terms of three healthcare indicators:[47]

1   Healthcare quality (Medicare plan ratings, quality of nursing homes and hospitals, and preventable hospital admissions).

Table 1.2

Spearman Rank Correlations among State Healthcare Ranking Indicators

Indicator	Healthcare Quality	Healthcare Access	Public Health Outcomes
Healthcare quality	—	0.45*	0.62*
Healthcare access	—	—	0.53*
Public health outcomes	—	—	—

* r_s statistically significant at $P < 0.01$.
SOURCE: State healthcare ranking data from Zeigler (2019).[47]

Table 1.3

Spearman Rank Correlations between State Healthcare Ranking Indicators and Upstream Metrics that Predict Health Outcomes

Metric	Healthcare Quality	Healthcare Access	Public Health Outcomes
Life expectancy at birth[24,25]	0.59*	0.66*	0.88*
Population happiness[48]	0.60*	0.52*	0.78*
Median family income[49]	0.56*	0.60*	0.73*
America's greenest states[49]	0.51*	0.74*	0.78*
Multiple study environmental index[49]	0.67*	0.60*	0.56*

* r_s statistically significant at $P < 0.01$.
SOURCE: State healthcare rankings from Zeigler (2019).[47]

2   Healthcare access (children or adults who do not have medical and dental care).
3   Public health outcomes (mental health, obesity, smoking, suicide, and mortality among adults and infants).

We compared the rankings across the three indicators and found them all statistically significantly correlated at $P < 0.01$ (Table 1.2). This finding is not surprising because health outcomes are statistically associated with access to high-quality health care. We then tested the hypothesis that these same indicators were also associated with the social, economic, and environmental metrics that predict health outcomes: life expectancy at birth,[24,25] population happiness (a surrogate for mental and social health),[48] median family income,[49] "green state" rankings,[49] and a multiple study environmental index[49] (Table 1.3). The Spearman rank-order correlations in Table 1.3 fall between 0.88 and 0.51, all statistically significant at $P < 0.01$.

Table 1.4

U.S. States with the Highest and Lowest Healthcare Rankings, 2019

State	Healthcare Quality	Healthcare Access	Public Health Outcomes
Highest ranked			
1. Hawaii	1	3	4
2. Massachusetts	13	2	5
3. Connecticut	14	1	6
4. Washington	3	12	9
5. Rhode Island	9	6	19
Lowest ranked			
46. Alabama	39	37	47
47. Oklahoma	46	48	45
48. West Virginia	48	28	50
49. Arkansas	49	45	49
50. Mississippi	50	50	48

SOURCE: Data abstracted from Ziegler (2019).[47]

The strongest association was between life expectancy at birth and public health outcomes, a finding that is not terribly surprising. Next, population happiness and America's greenest state metrics were tied in the strength of association with public health outcomes. This may not surprise readers who are familiar with the general observation that the more environmentally progressive states tend to have stronger economies, stronger environmental programs, and happier people. If there is a surprise, it is with the significant correlations between the three *US News & World Report* indicators and the multiple-study environmental index developed by Greenberg and Schneider[49] using state data over the last half-century. In summary, the data show that several social and environmental metrics are clearly associated with healthcare quality, healthcare access, and public health outcomes.

Inherent in the above analysis is the general pattern of health inequities across the fifty states. Table 1.4 highlights these by comparing the five states with the highest healthcare quality in the year 2019 *U.S. News & World Report* survey with those with the five lowest rankings. We should not take these rankings at face value, but they do show consistent differences across the states in health outcomes and the factors frequently associated with them.

In 1990, the average life expectancy at birth in the five states with the highest healthcare quality was 77.1 years, compared with 74.1 years in the five states with the lowest healthcare quality, a difference of three years. In

2016, the difference increased to 3.4 years as the life expectancy in the two sets of states increased to 80.5 and 75.4 years, respectively.[25]

For the United States as a whole, life expectancy increased to over the sixty years before 2014, reaching a zenith of 78.87 years then declining slightly for the three years after that. Woolf and Schoomaker[50] reported that the decline was driven primarily by increased midlife mortality from drug overdoses, alcohol abuse, suicides, and organ system diseases, particularly in New England and the Ohio Valley. They called for developing an understanding of the underlying causes because the implications for both public health and the overall economy are substantial. Life expectancy for 2020 was reported at 78.93, but it did not account for the impact of COVID-19.[51]

Healthcare Cost Imperative

This book does not focus on healthcare costs. However, it would be naive to assume that increasing healthcare costs should not concern us all. It is equally important to recognize that poor people living in poor places are less likely to have access to effective health care. With those caveats noted, in 1960 healthcare costs were 5 percent of U.S. gross domestic product (GDP). In 1980, the number increased to 8.9 percent, and the average healthcare expenditure per capita exceeded $1,100. By that time, the United States had higher healthcare costs per capita than did twelve other countries similar in development and wealth (Australia, Canada, Denmark, France, Germany, Japan, New Zealand, Norway, Sweden, Switzerland, the Netherlands, and the United Kingdom). In 2012, per capita expenditures on health care in the United States reached $8,745 (17.3 percent of GDP). In comparison, the average of the other twelve countries was $4,504 (10.6 percent of GDP). In 2019, health care was estimated to be 17.8 percent of GDP, with the gap between U.S. expenditures and those of other developed nations still growing.[52,53]

Various explanations have been offered for this growing issue with cost. Some of these explanations do not seem to stand the test of scrutiny. For example, the charge that the United States has an older population is not true, nor is the assertion that our healthcare system is more accessible and people use healthcare more than they do in other countries. Similarly, the statement that our healthcare system provides higher quality care is also highly debatable. On the other hand, there are explanations that seem to be consistent with reality. For instance, the United States has higher cost procedures and technology available for diagnosis and treatment, and we charge much higher prices for those luxuries. In addition, a large proportion of our population is uninsured, so when they seek medical care it is in settings that are more expensive. Lastly, our national performance at preventing disease leaves a lot to be desired.[54-57]

As much as Americans are troubled by the increase in healthcare costs, many are equally distressed by the failure of the United States to have the best health outcomes. For example, the U.S. Central Intelligence Agency's *World Factbook*[58] reported life expectancy at birth for the United States and the twelve countries we previously discussed. Japan had the highest life expectancy at 85.3 years. The average for all twelve comparison countries was 81.8 years. However, in the United States life expectancy was 80.0 years—lower than eleven of the twelve comparison countries. Reporting for the Global Burden of Disease Study, Foreman and colleagues[59] noted that the United States ranked 43rd in life expectancy in 2016, and that forecasting models put it at 64th by the year 2040. By contrast, fifty-nine countries (including China) were projected to surpass a life expectancy of eighty years by 2040. Those at the top of the life expectancy ranks were

1 Spain—85.8 years
2 Japan—85.7 years
3 Singapore—85.4 years
4 Switzerland—85.2 years
5 Portugal—84.5 years
6 Italy—84.5 years
7 Israel—84.4 years
8 France—84.3 years
9 Luxembourg—84.1 years
10 Australia—84.1 years

The current data and the forecasts for life expectancy in the United States in 2040 do not paint a rosy picture. The nation is clearly failing to achieve high-quality, long lives compared with other developed nations, and the costs incurred have led many to question whether the United States is on the wrong path in its provision of health care.

The Kaiser Family Foundation (KFF) has been tracking public reaction to healthcare costs and accomplishments. A January 2019 report shows how the issue both confuses many residents and has taken on a clear partisan perspective.[58] On December 14, 2018, a federal district court judge in Texas ruled the Affordable Care Act of 2010 (ACA) invalid. While the legal case proceeded, the KFF measured public reaction to the ruling. We focus on two notable findings. Fewer than half of the public was aware of the judge's ruling or understood it to rule against ACA. Overall, 41 percent of Americans approved the judge's ruling (81 percent of Republicans, 16 percent of Democrats, and 44 percent of independents). Even more fascinating was that respondents often dramatically changed their views after being told how the ruling would influence protections for pre-existing conditions and young adults. For example, after hearing that people with existing health conditions would have to pay more for coverage or could be denied coverage altogether, the 41 percent overall approval rating fell to 13 percent. When told that young adults would no longer be able to stay on their parents' insurance plans until age twenty-six, overall approval fell to 8 percent.

The survey also reviewed the public's attitude about the proposal to expand Medicare and Medicaid. Concerning a national health plan (Medicare for All), 56 percent of respondents favored the idea. By comparison, about 75 percent favored allowing people between fifty and sixty-four to purchase health insurance through Medicare, allowing people who do not get health insurance at work to buy health insurance through their state Medicaid program, and/or creating a national government-administered health plan similar to Medicare open to everyone. These responses changed when people learned additional information about possible delays with getting some medical tests and treatments, the possibility that most Americans would pay more in taxes, and so on. In other words, the public has a basic partisan perspective on healthcare policies, but their collective viewpoint is clearly subject to change based on what they are told or not told about the implications of changing policies.

Health in All Policies and the Culture of Health

Increasing both human health and quality of life are ultimate professional and personal goals for many who will read this book. Some places within the United States made sustained progress in improving the health of their populations for decades. Others have made much less progress, and a few even had reversals. As a nation, we should want to accomplish the following:

- Influence individual physical, mental, and social processes that cumulatively affect health.
- Improve access to preventative and curative health care.
- Improve the quality of science to be able to detect and address the physical, mental, and social determinants of health.

A concerted effort by the federal and state governments to increase access to quality care surely would help. However, it is just as likely that the U.S. government and selected states will decrease the resources needed to increase public access to health care, particularly in this time of economic strain and budget deficits. Similarly, some corporations hope to decrease worker healthcare-related costs by shifting premiums and co-pays directly to workers.

Given this cost-cutting environment, two ideas for improving the overall health of the public that are not directly linked to healthcare costs have been championed by some state governments and not-for-profit organizations. The first of these ideas is Health in All Policies (HiAP).[60,61] The state of California, the American Public Health Association, and the Public Health Institute chose to focus specifically on HiAP.[59] In New Jersey, the Bloustein School at Rutgers University provides HiAP training through the Planning Healthy Communities Initiative (PHCI).[62] These entities recognize the growing importance of local and state governments in improving public health by improving and increasing access to the upstream determinants of health, such as transportation, education, housing, healthy food, clean air, potable water, economic opportunity, open space, health care, libraries, financial services, energy, art and cultural opportunities, recreational environments, and opportunities for civic engagement.

A key objective of HiAP is to inform decision-makers about the health consequences of their policies, in particular those that bear upon:

- Equity—justice, or freedom from bias or favoritism.[63]
- Sustainability—using a resource so that it is not depleted or permanently damaged.[64]
- Resilience—the ability to recover from or adjust to change.[65]

Another key objective of HiAP is to involve multiple parties to jointly press for health considerations in the policy-making process. Using a university as an illustration, in the past advocacy and evidence for a health-related policy would likely come from a medical school, dental school, or school of public health. The HiAP agenda would seek input from departments of engineering, environmental science, geography, health administration, law, nutrition, public policy, social work, sociology, urban planning, and other academic units that directly or indirectly conduct research and provide services associated with health outcomes.

With regard to state and local government, HiAP means that staffers and commissioners who may rarely speak with one another will need to develop joint plans that they can live with. This will frankly be an uphill climb for some departments. In corporate settings, some of this kind of planning is already occurring, partly influenced by financial considerations and the need to build corporate resilience.[66] Single-issue nonprofit organizations will be hard-pressed to redirect their fundraising and advocacy toward a broader set of HiAP considerations. Only under the best of circumstances— meaning states with progressive leadership across both political parties— can we imagine strong state government engagement with HiAP across the United States.

The second idea for improving the overall health of the public, which is not directly linked to the cost of health care, is building a culture of health. This idea, we believe, is an even greater challenge for implementation than HiAP. For example, in 2015 Risa Lavizzo-Mourey, the president and CEO of the Robert Wood Johnson Foundation (RWJF) from 2003 to 2017, called for building a culture of health in the United States.[66] Her argument was that while progress has been made in public health, large inequities exist based on geography, ethnicity, and other factors: "Your ZIP code at birth may be as important as your medical load in predicting how long you live" (846).

Also in 2015, Alonzo Plough, the vice president for research evaluation learning and chief science officer at RWJF, made the case for a culture of health and provided support in the form of case studies in a special issue of the *American Journal of Public Health*.[67] Plough asserted that income, education, ethnicity, and where people live unequally influence the health of Americans. He states that too much emphasis remains on medical solutions and more needs focusing on social, environmental, economic, and other upstream determinants of health. Plough called for a nationwide, shared value that health is an action and policy priority. Drawing on social network theory, well-being science, community resilience, and community literature, Plough wants to build feelings of interdependence among people, places, and organizations around health. What this means is that hospitals, health departments, healthcare payors, governments, educational institutions, local community organizations, businesses, and individuals must work together as well as independently to focus attention on human health. This interconnected network of advocates, he believes, would then put the United States in a position to meet the dual objectives of improving health for the country as a whole and reducing health disparities.

We believe that accepting a culture of health as a priority in the United States would be a transformational change, one as important as the Social Transformation of American Medicine documented by Paul Starr.[68] Many interests and institutions will oppose this kind of rethinking, particularly those vested in the traditional medical model of health care. Nevertheless, RWJF is a powerful financial and political player in public health in the United States, and we believe that it will continue to invest heavily in order to fulfill its mission.

Charles Maurice de Talleyrand-Périgord was a mid-eighteenth-century French diplomat in the regime of Louis XVI. His statement that "whoever did not live in the years neighboring 1789 does not know what the pleasure of living means"[69] makes us think of the 1960s, when only 5 percent the U.S. GDP was related to health. There was, however, bipartisan support for policies such as Social Security, new housing, and other initiatives with public health implications. Since then, budget pressures have forced officials to make implicit and sometimes explicit decisions that adversely influence health outcomes.

HiAP and the culture of health are important for staving off the forces pushing a downward spiral of public health owing to trends in corruption, social and economic inequities, and the rapid spread of addiction, globalization, and other imposing trends. These rapidly escalating trends pose both risks and opportunities related to climate change, cybersecurity, financial risks, the spread of diseases, and other national and international challenges. Thus, we believe health has to be a core part of the debate as the United States, New Jersey, and local governments try to halt these runaway trains.

Organization of This Book

Chapter 2 begins with outsiders' perceptions of New Jersey, and it reviews measures of health in the state relative to those of other states. It examines the health disparities within New Jersey, including how the physical and historical environments of the state have shaped these outcomes. Finally, it reviews the role of government and the public in shaping New Jersey's health policies and overall public health.

Chapters 3, 4, and 5 cover the eras of movement to the "burbs," the baby boom generation, disparities and unrest, and the designation by the media of New Jersey as "Cancer Alley." Early on, there was great optimism about the nation's future, with the uncontrolled expansion of highways and suburbs, and a rise in middle-class consumerism. As white flight divided our cities and suburbs, the racial divide became increasingly apparent in housing and education as well as in access to and the delivery of healthcare services. By the 1970s, the public had become concerned about environmental and occupational exposures to toxins, particularly as the cause of cancer. The media found it easier to focus on these external causes of adverse health outcomes rather than offer alternative explanations, such as the role of smoking, diet, and alcohol-related behaviors. Chapter 4 discusses both the external and individual cancer risk factors that affected the state's many subpopulations during this period, particularly the health outcomes of our most vulnerable residents.

The 1980s saw a rise in gun violence, civil unrest, a crack epidemic along with threats from emerging infectious diseases such as HIV and acquired immunodeficiency syndrome (AIDS). We draw parallels to today's challenges, particularly with the COVID-19 pandemic that hit the nation, including the New York/New Jersey region, with explosive force. Chapter 5 briefly describes these historic challenges, focusing on the responses that involved science, education, and public policy decisions that reduced the risk from death and disease in New Jersey.

The 1990s were a time of significant economic upheaval in the United States. The loss of manufacturing jobs, efforts at urban redevelopment, and the failure of the suburban movement spurred efforts to achieve "Smart Growth." Chapter 6 discusses the repercussions of these economic shifts in both New Jersey and the nation as a whole. It also reviews the status of racial, ethnic, and income segregation during this period. The chapter focuses on the half-century-long legal and political struggle between the New Jersey Supreme Court and protectors of legislative prerogatives in home rule. The challenges over affordable housing and public school education both had major impacts on health outcomes.

By the end of the millennium, terrorism and natural hazards became the focus of public health across the nation. The September 11 and anthrax attacks of 2001 set the agenda for the public's concern about terrorism for many years. The increase in the ferocity of storms, including hurricanes that hit the state, brought about concerns for climate change. How New Jersey officials and the public reacted to these challenges is the focus of Chapter 7—particularly through hazard mitigation plans and actions. Also included are how fear and security measures influenced health care and health outcomes, and how those differed in New Jersey relative to the nation as a whole.

The reshuffling of health care is our focus in Chapter 8. The healthcare industry underwent massive consolidation during the second decade of the twenty-first century, and concerns about who pays and how to keep the system afloat became manifest. The chapter covers the increase in the availability of electronic medical records, changes in billing systems, and the costs of charity care, at both the state and the federal levels. The goal for the future of health care is to build a more cooperative set of relationships in which local health and local elected officials play a much more pivotal role in decisions about delivering health care and preventive health than in the past.

The epilogue examines seven challenges that threaten steady progress toward a healthier New Jersey during the next several decades: (1) pandemics and epidemics; (2) addictive behaviors; (3) coping with accelerated change and increased uncertainty; (4) cascading environmental threats; (5) growing disparities in economic, social, and political access; (6) demographic change; and (7) politics, power, and hedgehog and fox strategies. Each of these challenges may make it difficult to pursue a HiAP approach and build a broad culture of health, but we must try if we are to improve the health of our population over the next twenty-five years.

References

1   Grad FP. The preamble of the constitution of the World Health Organization. *Bull World Health Organ.* 2002;80(12):981–982.
2   Eberst RM. Defining health: a multidimensional model. *J Sch Health.* 1984;54(3): 99–104. doi:10.1111/j.1746-1561.1984.tb08780.x

3 Brüssow H. What is health? *Microb Biotechnol.* 2013;6(4):341–348. doi:10.1111/
1751-7915.12063

4 Bircher J, Kuruvilla S. Defining health by addressing individual, social, and
environmental determinants: new opportunities for health care and public health.
J Public Health Policy. 2014;35(3):363–386. doi:10.1057/jphp.2014.19

5 Ereshefsky M. Defining "health" and "disease." *Stud Hist Philos Biol Biomed Sci.*
2009;40(3):221–227. doi:10.1016/j.shpsc.2009.06.005

6 Public Health Service, Office of the Surgeon General. *Healthy People: The Surgeon
General's Report on Health Promotion and Disease Prevention.* DHEW (PHS) Pub
No. 79-55071. Washington, DC: U.S. Government Printing Office; 1979. https://
profiles.nlm.nih.gov/101584932X92

7 Public Health Service. *Promoting Health/Preventing Disease: Objectives for the
Nation.* Washington, DC: U.S. Government Printing Office; 1980. https://stacks
.cdc.gov/view/cdc/5293

8 Centers for Disease Control and Prevention. Health objectives for the nation.
MMWR Morb Mortal Wkly Rep. 1989;38(37):629–633. https://www.cdc.gov
/mmwr/preview/mmwrhtml/00001462.htm

9 Office of Disease Prevention and Health Promotion, Centers for Disease Control and
Prevention. Development of the National Health Promotion and Disease Prevention
Objectives for 2030. Updated February 6, 2022. https://www.healthypeople.gov/2020
/About-Healthy-People/Development-Healthy-People-2030

10 American Public Health Association. *Model Standards: Guide for Community
Preventive Health Services.* 2nd ed. Washington, DC: American Public Health
Association; 1985.

11 Office of Disease Prevention and Health Promotion, Centers for Disease Control
and Prevention. Healthy People 2010. [Archive] https://healthypeople.gov/2010/

12 Office of Disease Prevention and Health Promotion, Centers for Disease Control
and Prevention. Healthy People 2020. Updated February 6, 2022. https://www
.healthypeople.gov/2020/

13 Office of Disease Prevention and Health Promotion, Centers for Disease Control
and Prevention. Healthy People 2020: 2020 LHI topics. Updated February 6,
2022. https://www.healthypeople.gov/2020/leading-health-indicators/2020-LHI
-Topics

14 Bharmal N, Derose K, Felician M, Weden M. Understanding the upstream social
determinants of health. RAND Working Paper WR-1096-RC. May 2015. https://
www.rand.org/content/dam/rand/pubs/working_papers/WR1000/WR1096
/RAND_WR1096.pdf

15 Centers for Disease Control and Prevention. NCHHSTP social determinants of
health. Updated May 9, 2022. https://www.cdc.gov/nchhstp/socialdeterminants
/index.html

16 Link BG, Phelan J. Social conditions as fundamental causes of disease. *J Health
Soc Behav.* 1995;Spec No:80–94. https://drexel.edu/greatworks/Theme/Winter
/~/media/Files/greatworks/WI12/LinkandPhelan1995.ashx

17 Centers for Disease Control and Prevention. Developing Healthy People 2030.
Accessed September 1, 2022. https://health.gov/healthypeople

18 Gakidou E, Afshin A, Abajobir AA, et al. Global, regional, and national comparative risk assessment of 84 behavioural, environmental and occupational, and
metabolic risks or clusters of risks, 1990–2016: a systematic analysis for the Global

Burden of Disease Study 2016. *Lancet.* 2017;390(10100):1345–1422. doi:10.1016/S0140-6736(17)32366-8

19 Hay SI, Abajobir AA, Abate KH, et al. Global, regional, and national disability-adjusted life-years (DALYs) for 333 diseases and injuries and healthy life expectancy (HALE) for 195 countries and territories, 1990–2016: a systematic analysis for the Global Burden of Disease Study 2016. *Lancet.* 2017;390(10100):1260–1344. doi:10.1016/S0140-6736(17)32130-X

20 Vos T, Abajobir AA, Abate KH, et al. Global, regional, and national incidence, prevalence, and years lived with disability for 328 diseases and injuries for 195 countries, 1990–2016: a systematic analysis for the Global Burden of Disease Study 2016. *Lancet.* 2017;390(10100):1211–1259. doi:10.1016/S0140-6736(17)32154-2

21 Naghavi M, Abajobir AA, Abbafati C, et al. Global, regional, and national age-sex specific mortality for 264 causes of death, 1980–2016: a systematic analysis for the Global Burden of Disease Study 2016. *Lancet.* 2017;390(10100):1151–1210. doi:10.1016/S0140-6736(17)32152-9

22 Wang H, Abajobir AA, Abate KH, et al. Global, regional, and national under-5 mortality, adult mortality, age-specific mortality, and life expectancy, 1970–2016: a systematic analysis for the Global Burden of Disease Study 2016. *Lancet.* 2017;390(10100):1084–1150. doi:10.1016/S0140-6736(17)31833-0

23 Fullman N, Barber RM, Abajobir AA, et al. Measuring progress and projecting attainment on the basis of past trends of the health-related Sustainable Development Goals in 188 countries: an analysis from the Global Burden of Disease Study 2016. *Lancet.* 2017;390(10100):1423–1459. doi:10.1016/S0140-6736(17)32336-X

24 US Burden of Disease Collaborators, Mokdad AH, Ballestros K, et al. The state of US health, 1990–2016: burden of diseases, injuries, and risk factors among US states. *JAMA.* 2018;319(14):1444–1472. doi:10.1001/jama.2018.0158

25 Murray CJL, Atkinson C, Bhalla K, et al. The state of US health, 1990–2010: burden of diseases, injuries, and risk factors. *JAMA.* 2013;310(6):591–608. doi:10.1001/jama.2013.13805

26 Wu Y, Jin A, Xie G, et al. The 20 most important and most preventable health problems of China: a Delphi consultation of Chinese experts. *Am J Public Health.* 2018;108(12):1592–1598. doi:10.2105/AJPH.2018.304684

27 Mokdad AH, Bowman BA, Ford ES, Vinicor F, Marks JS, Koplan JP. The continuing epidemics of obesity and diabetes in the United States. *JAMA.* 2001;286(10):1195. doi:10.1001/jama.286.10.1195

28 Haskell WL, Lee I-M, Pate RR, et al. Physical activity and public health: updated recommendation for adults from the American College of Sports Medicine and the American Heart Association. *Circulation.* 2007;116(9):1081–1093. doi:10.1161/CIRCULATIONAHA.107.185649

29 Manyema M, Veerman LJ, Tugendhaft A, et al. Modelling the potential impact of a sugar-sweetened beverage tax on stroke mortality, costs and health-adjusted life years in South Africa. *BMC Public Health.* 2016;16(1):405. doi:10.1186/s12889-016-3085-y

30 Brown DW, Balluz LS, Giles WH, et al. Diabetes mellitus and health-related quality of life among older adults. *Diabetes Res Clin Pract.* 2004;65(2):105–115. doi:10.1016/j.diabres.2003.11.014

31 Urban LE, Roberts SB, Fierstein JL, et al. Sodium, saturated fat, and trans fat content per 1,000 kilocalories: temporal trends in fast-food restaurants, United States, 2000–2013. *Prev Chronic Dis*. 2014;11:E228. doi:10.5888/pcd11.140335

32 Mokdad AH, Ford ES, Bowman BA, et al. Prevalence of obesity, diabetes, and obesity-related health risk factors, 2001. *JAMA*. 2003;289(1):76–79. doi:10.1001/jama.289.1.76

33 Dalen JE, Alpert JS, Goldberg RJ, Weinstein RS. The epidemic of the 20th century: coronary heart disease. *Am J Med*. 2014;127(9):807–812. doi:10.1016/j.amjmed.2014.04.015

34 Dwyer-Lindgren L, Bertozzi-Villa A, Stubbs RW, et al. Inequalities in life expectancy among U.S. counties, 1980 to 2014: temporal trends and key drivers. *JAMA Intern Med*. 2017;177(7):1003–1011. doi:10.1001/jamainternmed.2017.0918

35 Micha R, Peñalvo JL, Cudhea F, et al. Association between dietary factors and mortality from heart disease, stroke, and type 2 diabetes in the United States. *JAMA*. 2017;317(9):912. doi:10.1001/jama.2017.0947

36 Case A, Deaton A. Mortality and morbidity in the 21st century. *Brookings Pap Econ Act*. 2017;2017:397–476. doi:10.1353/eca.2017.0005

37 National Institute on Drug Abuse (NIDA). Overdose death rates. Updated January 20, 2022. https://nida.nih.gov/research-topics/trends-statistics/overdose-death-rates

38 Harris RD. Suicide in the workplace. *Mon Labor Rev*. December 2016. doi:10.21916/mlr.2016.54

39 Miller M, Warren M, Hemenway D, Azrael D. Firearms and suicide in US cities. *Inj Prev*. 2015;21(e1):e116–e119. doi:10.1136/injuryprev-2013-040969

40 Miller M, Hemenway D. Guns and suicide in the United States. *N Engl J Med*. 2008;359(10):989–991. doi:10.1056/NEJMp0805923

41 Firneisz G. Non-alcoholic fatty liver disease and type 2 diabetes mellitus: the liver disease of our age? *World J Gastroenterol*. 2014;20(27):9072–9089. doi:10.3748/wjg.v20.i27.9072

42 Ortiz-Lopez C, Lomonaco R, Orsak B, et al. Prevalence of prediabetes and diabetes and metabolic profile of patients with nonalcoholic fatty liver disease (NAFLD). *Diabetes Care*. 2012;35(4):873–878. doi:10.2337/dc11-1849

43 Siegel M, Negussie Y, Vanture S, et al. The relationship between gun ownership and stranger and nonstranger firearm homicide rates in the United States, 1981–2010. *Am J Public Health*. 2014;104(10):1912–1919. doi:10.2105/AJPH.2014.302042

44 Li C, Ford ES, Zhao G, et al. Prevalence and correlates of undiagnosed depression among U.S. adults with diabetes: the Behavioral Risk Factor Surveillance System, 2006. *Diabetes Res Clin Pract*. 2009;83(2):268–279. doi:10.1016/j.diabres.2008.11.006

45 Vigdor ER, Mercy JA. Do laws restricting access to firearms by domestic violence offenders prevent intimate partner homicide? *Eval Rev*. 2006;30(3):313–346. doi:10.1177/0193841X06287307

46 Barna M. Experts fear suicide, deaths of despair will rise in wake of COVID-19: mental health crisis. *Nations Health*. 2020;50(5):1–10. https://www.thenationshealth.org/content/50/5/1.1

47 Ziegler B. Best States 2019: Health Care Rankings. *U.S. News & World Report*. Accessed September 12, 2021. https://web.archive.org/web/20190622180925/https://www.usnews.com/news/best-states/rankings/health-care

48 Bernardo R. 2017's Happiest states in America. *WalletHub*, September 11, 2017. https://web.archive.org/web/20171224074156/https://wallethub.com/edu/happiest-states/6959/

49 Greenberg MR, Schneider D. Environmental Health and the U.S. Federal System: Sustainably Managing Health Hazards. UK: Routledge; 2019. https://www.taylorfrancis.com/books/mono/10.4324/9780429264757/environmental-health-federal-system-michael-greenberg-dona-schneider

50 Woolf SH, Schoomaker H. Life expectancy and mortality rates in the United States, 1959–2017. *JAMA*. 2019;322(20):1996. doi:10.1001/jama.2019.16932

51 U.S. Life Expectancy 1950–2020. MacroTrends. Accessed August 26, 2020. https://www.macrotrends.net/countries/USA/united-states/life-expectancy

52 Mikulic M. U.S. national health expenditure as percent of GDP 1960–2019. *Statista*, August 9, 2019. https://web.archive.org/web/20191218203728/https://www.statista.com/statistics/184968/us-health-expenditure-as-percent-of-gdp-since-1960/

53 Mikulic M. Health expenditure as a percentage of GDP in select countries 2018. *Statista*, November 12, 2019. https://web.archive.org/web/20191114171612/https://www.statista.com/statistics/268826/health-expenditure-as-gdp-percentage-in-oecd-countries/

54 Commins J. Healthcare spending at 20% of GDP? That's an economy-wide problem. *HealthLeaders*, September 19, 2018. https://www.healthleadersmedia.com/finance/healthcare-spending-20-gdp-thats-economy-wide-problem

55 Woolhandler S, Campbell T, Himmelstein DU. Costs of health care administration in the United States and Canada. *N Engl J Med*. 2003;349(8):768–775. doi:10.1056/NEJMsa022033

56 Bodenheimer T. High and rising health care costs. Part 1: seeking an explanation. *Ann Intern Med*. 2005;142(10):847–854. doi:10.7326/0003-4819-142-10-200505170-00010

57 Bodenheimer T. High and rising health care costs. Part 2: technologic innovation. *Ann Intern Med*. 2005;142(11):932–937. doi:10.7326/0003-4819-142-11-200506070-00012

58 U.S. Central Intelligence Agency. *The World Factbook,* 2019. https://www.cia.gov/the-world-factbook/

59 Foreman KJ, Marquez N, Dolgert A, et al. Forecasting life expectancy, years of life lost, and all-cause and cause-specific mortality for 250 causes of death: reference and alternative scenarios for 2016–40 for 195 countries and territories. *Lancet*. 2018;392(10159):2052–2090. doi:10.1016/S0140-6736(18)31694-5

60 Rudolph L, Caplan J, Ben-Moshe K, Dillon L. *Health in All Policies: A Guide for State and Local Governments*. Washington, DC: American Public Health Association and Public Health Institute; 2013. https://www.apha.org/-/media/Files/PDF/factsheets/Health_inAll_Policies_Guide_169pages.ashx

61 Benjamin GC, Troutman A. *An Introduction to Health in All Policies: A Guide for State and Local Governments*. Washington, DC: American Public Health Association and Public Health Institute; 2013. http://www.phi.org/wp-content/uploads/migration/uploads/files/Four_Pager_Health_in_All_Policies-A_Guide_for_State_and_Local_Governments.pdf

62 Planning Healthy Communities Initiative. Accessed June 20, 2022. http://phci.rutgers.edu

63 Equity. In: Merriam-Webster.com Dictionary. Accessed September 12, 2021. https://www.merriam-webster.com/dictionary/equity

64 Sustainability. In: Merriam-Webster.com Dictionary. Accessed September 12, 2021. https://www.merriam-webster.com/dictionary/sustainability

65 Resilience. In: Merriam-Webster.com Dictionary. Accessed September 12, 2021. https://www.merriam-webster.com/dictionary/resilience

66 Kunreuther H, Useem M. *Mastering Catastrophic Risk: How Companies Are Coping with Disruption*. New York: Oxford University Press; 2018.

67 Plough AL. Building a culture of health: a critical role for public health services and systems research. *Am J Public Health*. 2015;105(Suppl 2):S150–S152. doi:10.2105/AJPH.2014.302410

68 Starr P. *The Social Transformation of American Medicine: The Rise of a Sovereign Profession and the Making of a Vast Industry*. New York: Basic Books; 1982.

69 Life. In: Hoyt JK, Roberts KL, comps. *Hoyt's New Cyclopedia of Practical Quotations*. New York: Funk & Wagnalls; 1922. Bartleby.com; 2009. https://www.bartleby.com/78/

2

The Winding Path
to Better Health
in New Jersey

───────────────●───────────────

We start this chapter with a reality check about public perceptions of New Jersey and the health of its residents, primarily those held by people who live outside the state. These perceptions are often out of touch with reality. Thus, this chapter has five objectives:

1 Summarize outsiders' perceptions of New Jersey.
2 Examine metrics used to measure health in New Jersey compared with other states.
3 Examine metrics used to measure health within the diverse populations who live in New Jersey.
4 Consider the physical and historical environments of New Jersey and how these have helped shape the state's evolution and its health outcomes.
5 Review the role of government and the public in shaping health policies for New Jersey.

Introduction to the Garden State

New Jersey is a small state of 8,700 square miles. It ranks 47 out of the fifty states in size but ranks 11 in population (with >9 million residents). One of the state's well-known attributes is that it is the only state with a population density of more than 1,000 people per square mile. Being a densely populated state is typically associated with high automobile traffic, crowding, and noise—perceptions we cannot deny, at least for many parts of the state. On the other hand, New Jersey's racial and ethnic diversity is less well-known, which some welcome and others do not. Also, New Jersey is among the most affluent states, in recent years ranking first, second, or third in median household income, a fact that many outsiders fail to appreciate or choose to ignore.

As Peter Moore, working for YouGov, opined in a 2015 article, "New Jersey is the only state which Americans tend to have an unfavorable opinion of."[1] Moore reported that 40 percent of Americans have an unfavorable opinion of New Jersey while 30 percent have a favorable opinion of the state. This yields a net favorability rating of minus 10 percent. (The second least popular state listed in that opinion piece was Alabama, but it had a net favorable rating of 8 percent.) As New Jersey residents, we must say that it was distressing to see the map of favorable states with New Jersey the only one in red (see chapter 4 for a similarly distressing story). By contrast, the most favorable state rating was achieved by Hawaii, with a net favorability rating of 56 percent. Other states with favorability ratings above 40 percent included Alaska, Maine, Montana, and Wyoming. From these ratings, it seems clear that, in at least in the YouGov survey, Americans prefer mountainous states.

Moore asserted that New Jersey epitomizes northeastern suburbia and that the popular image of the state often falls between the award-winning HBO crime drama *The Sopranos* and the MTV reality show *Jersey Shore*.[1] He also said that many people's views of New Jersey (see chapter 3) are strongly influenced by the gray industrial landscape that stretches along the upper reaches of the New Jersey Turnpike. Moore also added that those who live in New Jersey (New Jerseyans) tend to take a "hard-nosed attitude towards life," seeking out challenging circumstances and sacrificing leisure time to get ahead in their careers.

One response to Moore's review is to ignore it because our state's residents have heard it all before. Jennifer Legra's response to the maligning of New

Jersey is one we would expect from an annoyed and sarcastic state resident.[2] She gently summarizes New Jersey's contributions to sports, technology, and the Revolutionary War, then points to our many state parks and beaches, strong schools, and safety record. She also brags that a 2014 report picked two New Jersey cities, including the one she lives in, as among the top 10 safest cities in America (spoiler alert: Edison and Woodbridge Township). Regarding the state's location between New York City and Philadelphia, Legra adds,

> Who would want to be nestled between New York City and Philadelphia? Bleh. Awful places full of culture and history and world-famous cheesesteaks. And the nearby options when you live in New Jersey are countless: the beach, skiing, mountains, and city life. So many damn options—who needs 'em. Stupid New Jersey.[2]

To address education, she added,

> According to the Science and Engineering Readiness Index, New Jersey ranks the third highest state in Math and Science. What the f . . . Science and Math? As if those subjects matter these days. According to another dumb report released by EdWeek, New Jersey public education system ranks 3rd, among the best in the nation. Ugh! And, wait—get this—this year, New Jersey ranked second in the "Chance for Success" index and second in the number of students scoring at the advanced level on the National Assessment of Educational Progress. Then, it ranked third in K-12 achievement and has consistently ranked in the top 10 nationally on the report. Could you believe that garbage? Top 3? What a bunch of dummies.[2]

Without doubt, Legra's points about New Jersey are fun to read, but these are hardly unbiased. Monmouth University's April 2022 poll of state residents reports that 64 percent of respondents rated the state as excellent or good place to live (19 percent excellent, 45 percent as good). Yet, 22 percent rated it as fair and another 13 percent said poor. These results are a slight improvement over 2021 when 59 percent rated it as excellent or good. For context, the all-time low was 50 percent in February 2019 when the COVID pandemic was just beginning to become apparent. In February 1987, the rate of excellent and good ratings was 87 percent.[3]

We have found hundreds of comments about New Jersey from nonresidents and former residents. Here are few from Quora that have been trimmed to save space.[4]

- NONRESIDENT: "New Jersey has the disadvantage of being located right next to New York so it gets to bear the brunt of jokes made by New Yorkers about many things that would apply to the rest of the country and even more suburban parts of New York City itself. Many people have also only driven on the New Jersey Turnpike or flew to New York City through Newark Airport and as a result have only seen many of the least flattering parts of the state. If you look at any objective measure New Jersey has among the highest standards of living in the entire country."
- NONRESIDENT (NEW YORK): Jersey is honestly kind of a hidden gem. There was a Quora question awhile back, something like "of all the states you've been to, which one surprised you most?" I said New Jersey.
- Because it's so small and so crowded (#1 in the United States in population density), there's a tendency to think of Jersey as nothing but cities, factories, and featureless suburbs, with a coastline. And in much of northeastern Jersey, that's pretty much the way it is, honestly. But much of the rest of the state is quite lovely. A lot of northwest Jersey, like Warren County, is bucolic and peaceful, with small communities and a lot of friendly people.
- Pinelands National Reserve, which encompasses much of the southern half of the state, is a region of tremendous beauty and biodiversity, and was our first national reserve here in the United States. Within the reserve are the Pine Barrens, which have their own haunting beauty. The fine white sand beaches of Absecon Island are fabulous, and Cape May and Long Beach Island are paradises for beach bums in summer.
- My brother lives in that area, around midway between Philadelphia and Atlantic City, and in his rural little town, you'd never know you were in the most densely populated state in the union. So, I like Jersey. I kind of think of it as that annoying little sibling that you like to give a hard time to, but also have tremendous affection for and whose back you'll always have when the chips are down.

- FORMER RESIDENT: All those who are thinking of leaving New Jersey for "a better place to live" THINK AND THINK AGAIN! Appreciate what you have. The people who live in other states do not have life nearly as good as the love for you to think! You will cry to come home and not be able to someday! Heaven knows I did!

A final perception element is the ongoing tug-of-war for power between the northern and southern parts of the state. Writing in 1981, Bernardo considers the arguments made by southern New Jersey counties for succession from the state as a whole.[5] He notes that Brendan Byrne, then governor, reduced home rule power in New Jersey in order to make decisions that the governor felt were in the best interests of the entire state. One of these decisions was to back the redevelopment of Atlantic City. Another was the rejection of a proposed new highway to the New Jersey shore (see chapter 3). Additional political decisions helped fuel the southern New Jersey secessionist movement, but there is also the reality that a cultural discomfort exists between the southern and northern parts of the state. These differences play out in the prevalence of health risk factors and the resultant health outcomes, which we see when we examine health data at the county level. For example, striking differences can be seen in overall health outcomes from the more sparsely populated southern New Jersey counties in comparison with the more developed northern ones (Figure 2.1).[6]

Health in New Jersey Compared with the Nation: Before COVID-19

It is reasonable to assume that a state with negative outside perceptions would not attract people who have the option to select where they want to live. They would likely avoid places that they perceive would provide a low quality of life. However, basic findings show that the population of the state as a whole consider themselves happy and healthy. New Jerseyans simply live longer and with fewer disabilities compared with those in many other states. They are less likely to be obese, have high blood pressure, or have other chronic problems that predispose populations to a lower quality of life and premature mortality. The New Jersey population as a whole is also more affluent and more educated compared with the residents of many other

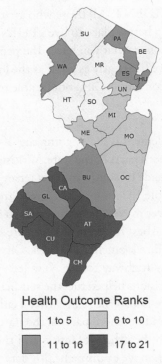

Health Outcome Ranks

□	1 to 5	▨	6 to 10
▨	11 to 16	■	17 to 21

FIGURE 2.1 Overall health outcome rankings by county, New Jersey 2020 (based on 2016–2018 data). (*Source:* University of Wisconsin Population Health Institute, New Jersey 2020, County Health Rankings & Roadmaps.[6])

states, thus predisposing them to have a high quality of life compared with Americans as a whole.

We combine data from 1990, 2016, and 2020 (before the COVID-19 pandemic) in the following summary. In 1990, New Jersey was at or close to the midpoint rank of the fifty states with regard to life expectancy at birth, healthy life expectancy at birth, age-standardized death rates, and metrics of premature death and disability (ranked 24th to 29th). By 2016, the New Jersey population showed improvements in almost every metric. For example, not only did life expectancy and healthy life expectancy at birth increase, but also New Jersey's ranks improved to 8 and 10, respectively, among the fifty states. Rates for premature death (seventh lowest among the states) and disabilities also improved, although the latter was not among the top 10.

Using a standardized data set prepared by the University of Wisconsin,[6] Tables 2.1 to 2.3 summarize New Jersey's health metrics in the year 2020

Table 2.1

Health Outcome Metrics for New Jersey and the United States, 2020, before COVID-19

Metric	United States	New Jersey	Lowest County in NJ	Highest County in NJ
Years of life lost before age 75 per 100,000 population (age-adjusted)	6,900	5,900	3,800	10,200
Live births <2,500 grams (low birthweight)	8%	8%	6%	10%
Report "poor" or "fair health (age-adjusted)	17%	18%	11%	24%
Report poor physical health days during last 30 days (age-adjusted)	3.8	3.7	2.8	4.4
Personal poor mental health days during last 30 days (age-adjusted)	4.0	3.9	3.4	4.7

SOURCE: University of Wisconsin Population Health Institute. New Jersey 2020. County Health Rankings & Roadmaps.[6]

compared with the United States as a whole for thirty-four commonly used metrics. Table 2.1 shows that New Jersey has an outcome profile similar to the nation as a whole. For loss of life before age seventy-five, it has a much better rate than the nation as a whole, which we believe is a strong indicator of upstream and downstream health indicator influence.

Table 2.2 shows some of the key behaviors that should lead to better future health outcomes: lower rates of births by teenage mothers, lower rates of sexually transmitted diseases, less evidence of excessive alcohol consumption and smoking, better food environments, and more access to exercise sites. Only in the case of self-reported physical inactivity does New Jersey have a weaker record. New Jersey is about the same as the nation in access to and use of clinical care services.

Table 2.3 presents social and environmental population-based indicators. New Jersey has better metrics for social indicators than the nation as a whole but not for environmental ones. Several of the latter reflect the reality of a densely developed state with wide variations among populations.

The last set of New Jersey-United States health comparisons appears in Table 2.4. *U.S. News and World Report* data casts New Jersey in a positive light with regard to crime and corrections, education, opportunity, the natural environment. The ranks are lower for the economy, fiscal stability, infrastructure, and transportation. The Gallup poll is strongest in reporting

Table 2.2

Health Behaviors and Clinical Care Indicators for New Jersey and the United States, 2020, before COVID-19

Metric	United States	New Jersey	Lowest County in NJ	Highest County in NJ
Health behaviors				
Births per 1,000 female population ages 15 to 19 years	23	13	2	16
Rate of sexually transmitted infections: newly diagnosed *Chlamydia* cases per 100,000 population	524.6	391.3	160.2	750.2
Adults reporting binge or heavy drinking	19%	18%	16%	22%
Driving deaths involving alcohol	28%	22%	13%	39%
Adult population currently smoking	17%	14%	11%	18%
Population ≥20 years with a body mass index ≥30 kg/m^2	29%	26%	20%	37%
Food environment index—factors contributing to a healthy food environment (0 = worst; 10 = best)	7.6	9.3	7.4	9.5
Adults reporting no leisure-time physical activity	23%	26%	19%	31%
Adults with access to exercise opportunities	84%	95%	70%	100%
Clinical care metrics				
Population <65 years with no insurance	10%	9%	5%	13%
Fee-for-service Medicare enrollees who had an annual flu vaccination	46%	49%	37%	48%
Medicare enrollees ages 65 to 74 years who received an annual mammography screening	42%	41%	34%	48%
Preventable hospital stays: hospital stays for ambulatory-care sensitive conditions per 100,000 Medicare enrollees	4,535	4,535	2,916	7,580
Ratio of population to primary care physicians	1,330:1	1,190:1	2,990:1	830:1
Ratio of population to dentists	1,450:1	1,160:1	2,980:1	770:1
Ratio of population to mental health providers	400:1	450:1	1,570:1	150:1

SOURCE: University of Wisconsin Population Health Institute. New Jersey 2020. County Health Rankings & Roadmaps.[6]

New Jersey's social and personal health indicators, but much less so for economic and community indicators.

The positive rankings in both the *U.S. News* and Gallup surveys, we believe, reflect the state's investment in social, educational, and environmental programs. A 1991 survey is illustrative in this regard. Hall and Kerr

Table 2.3

Social and Environmental Influences for New Jersey and the United States, 2020, before COVID-19

Metric	United States	New Jersey	Lowest County in NJ	Highest County in NJ
Social influences				
High school graduation within four years	85%	91%	81%	96%
Adults ages 25 to 44 years with some postsecondary education	66%	69%	40%	82%
Population ≥16 years who are unemployed but seeking employment	3.9%	4.1%	3.3%	8.4%
Population <18 years of age in poverty	18%	14%	4%	22%
Ratio of household income 80th percentile to 20th percentile	4.9	5.2	3.8	6.8
Children in single-parent households	33%	29%	14%	50%
Number of membership associations per 10,000 population	9.3	8.5	5.0	13.4
Reported violent crime offenses per 100,000 population	386	253	42	606
Injury deaths per 100,000 population	70	56	40	94
Physical environment influences				
Air pollution: Average daily density of PM 2.5	8.6	9.9	7.8	11.6
Households with at least one of the following problems: overcrowding, high costs, lack of kitchen facilities, or lack of plumbing	18%	22%	14%	31%
Drive alone to work	76%	71%	37%	85%
Long commute—driving alone	36%	43%	24%	58%

SOURCE: University of Wisconsin Population Health Institute. New Jersey 2020. County Health Rankings & Roadmaps.[6]

examined 256 environmental indicators, ranking the state third in state policy initiatives behind California and Oregon.[10] It would be a stretch to rank New Jersey that same level in 2020 because the state's environmental department now works with considerably fewer resources than it did then. The same conclusion can be reached about New Jersey's efforts in social, healthcare, educational, and community programs.

Cuts in state environmental programs have not only been for political agendas for over a decade, but they also reflect some economic realities. During the last decade, the state's economy suffered slow growth, and the state became embattled with unions regarding pensions. Currently, the economic impact of COVID-19 is painful and continues to impact quality of life.

Table 2.4
Health-Related Indicators and Rankings for New Jersey among the 50 U.S. States

Indicator	Rank of 50
Overall[7]	12
Health care (overall)[7]	6
• Access	13
• Quality	19
• Public health	3
Crime and corrections[7]	6
Economy[7]	31
Education[7]	2
Fiscal stability[7]	49
Infrastructure[7]	34
Opportunity[7]	8
Transportation (overall)[7]	38
• Commuter time	48
• Public transit use	2
• Road quality	46
• Bridge quality	29
Natural environment[7]	13
Well-being (overall)[8]	31
• Career	41
• Social	9
• Financial	28
• Community	40
• Physical	19
2018's happiest states in America[9]	13

SOURCES: U.S. News & World Report (2019);[7] Gallup (2019);[8] World Population Review (2018).[9]

Consequently, the fact that New Jersey's economy, fiscal stability, and infrastructure ratings are currently relatively low comes as no surprise, and COVID-19 only complicates the challenge.

The transportation rating, which we have broken up into categories, speaks to the current fiscal difficulty reflected in transportation. Overall, New Jersey ranked 38 of the fifty states for transportation. However, embedded within that overall ranking are four transportation metrics: commuter time (rank 48), public transit use (rank 2), road quality (rank 46), and bridge quality (rank 29). From these rankings, we conclude that New Jersey residents heavily rely on public transit, yet they appear chronically distressed by how long it takes to get to work. The low commuter time ignores the reality that

New Jersey has an extensive and ongoing commitment to public transit. The major reason why the state's transit system is chronically stressed is the steep reduction in federal financial support, with those in Washington preferring to have the states absorb as much of these costs as possible. In less politically contentious times, the federal and state governments worked together. However, the current state of affairs is marked by high levels of political contention, and these play out in reduced services designed to support the public's health and well-being (see chapters 3 and the epilogue for more detail).

The 2019 Gallup poll[8] rankings in Table 2.4 include an overall metric called well-being. New Jersey scores well in social well-being and reasonably well in physical well-being. Its low scores for career, financial, and community reflect, we believe, distress about balancing the state budget, the burden of taxes, and the types of services that are provided by the state. The overall well-being rank for New Jersey of 31 is a relatively weak score.

World Population Review[9] and earlier Bernardo[11] ranked the fifty states in overall happiness, including emotional and physical well-being scores and work environment indicators. The overall happiness rank for New Jersey was 13 compared with an overall well-being rank of 31 in the Gallup poll.[8] Some of the differences in ranking may have to do with the fact that the work environment questions in the two surveys have different wording. Additionally, political arguments around the economy and taxes are particularly strong at this time. Indeed, Bernardo's survey[11] had New Jersey ranked 6 in happiness, along with the lowest scores for suicides and depression. In the midst of the COVID-19 epidemic and many other tough challenges, "happiness" has taken a hit, but this same disaster has hit many other places. The first author, Michael Greenberg, contracted the disease as well but finds being alive and able to complete this book is a source of happiness. We acknowledge that the ability of others to engage in activities that make them happy has been disrupted, and it will take time to find a new normal level for happiness.

The COVID-19 Impact

The first COVID-19-related death in New Jersey was on March 10, 2020.[12] A little over a year later, on April 26, 2021, the toll stood at over 23,000 confirmed deaths.[13] One way of looking at these numbers is that New Jersey's death rate in 2020 was the highest in seventy-five years—that is, since 1945. In fact, 2020 was the first time since 1953 that more than 1 percent of the state's population died.[14] Yates asserts that the numbers of COVID-related deaths are even higher than reported because some people died at home from diabetes, Alzheimer's, and other causes that were triggered by COVID-19.[15]

Although mortality from the virus is important, so is morbidity—the ability of the virus to turn the economy upside down because of hospitalizations, work and school absences, the closing of businesses and the loss of jobs, and impediments to the simple ability of people to carry on with their lives. Morbidity, or the number of people sickened from COVID-19, continues to be significant in New Jersey, as documented by the number cases confirmed by viral and antigen tests. For example, on April 26, 2021, the number of confirmed cases in the state was the highest in the nation.[14]

New Jersey, along with New York City, was among the first areas in the United States hit by the virus,[16] and knowledge of what to do about the infection was limited (see chapter 7). Why was this region hit first? Both New Jersey and New York City are international air transportation hubs and rail hubs. As infected individuals entered the region through the hubs, the high population and job density in both areas greatly increased the probability of contact with infected individuals.[17] Furthermore, those at highest risk, seniors living in group housing, were hard to protect.[18,19]

To summarize, COVID-19 interrupted the slow and steady progress that New Jersey had been making toward a healthier state. In addition to the health, social, and economic burdens associated with COVID-19, the virus hurt the state's image as much as the Cancer Alley label did in the 1970s. There is legitimate concern about the economic and social health of New Jersey in light of COVID-19 and its variants. Yet the reality we see is that the attributes that led New Jersey to the path it was on before COVID-19 will reassert themselves as they did in the 1970s. We expect the threat will reinvigorate the population back toward its healthier path.

Differences in Health among New Jersey's Populations

Differences in the indicators of health among the states are revealing. However, we recognize that often much larger differences are found within the same political entity. The state of New Jersey has long collected data sets on more than 250 health-associated metrics—from 1,3-butadiene in outdoor air to youth suicide attempts. The state has prepared summary reports of the data sets collected, and researchers may request special calculations. Some data sets

Table 2.5

Selected Public Health Indicators by Categories of Residents, New Jersey, 2014 to 2016

Indicator	Health (Good, Very Good, Excellent), %	Age-Adjusted Death Rate per 100,000	Obesity[a]	Current Smoker[b]	Binge Drinking[c]	Influenza Vaccine in Past 12 Months, 65+ Years	Asthma Prevention, 18+ Years
Education, population 25+ years							
< High school	63.0	NA	34.2	20.6	11.8	NA	NA
High school grad or GED	80.3	NA	31.1	21.6	15.2	NA	NA
Some post–high school	84.7	NA	28.4	15.7	18.7	NA	NA
College grad	92.4	NA	19.8	7.3	16.1	NA	NA
Race/ethnicity							
White	87.1	700.3	24.9	16.0	17.6	62.1	7.6
Black	79.0	828.9	38.0	19.4	12.9	52.7	12.3
Hispanic	70.9	455.6	31.7	12.4	13.1	54.6	8.7
Asian	91.8	295.9	9.4	7.4	10.1	NA	5.3
Age							
18 to 34 years	90.1	NA	19.1	15.9	26.2	NA	8.0
35 to 49 years	86.1	NA	28.7	16.3	18.2	NA	7.6
50 to 64 years	79.1	NA	31.6	15.4	13.9	NA	8.7
65+ years	75.7	NA	27.5	8.4	5.7	60.2	7.7

Abbreviations: GED, general equivalency diploma; NA, not available.

SOURCE: Center for Health Statistics and Informatics, New Jersey State Health Assessment Data (NJSHAD), New Jersey Department of Health.[22]

[a] Defined as the percentage of adults with a body mass index ≥ 30 kg/m^2 (self-reported height and weight).

[b] Defined as adult 18+ years who smoke cigarettes every day or on some days.

[c] Adults 18+ reported binger drinking during the last 30 days before survey (5+ drinks for men and 4 for women).

are gathered every year, and others are collected only sporadically. The most complete set of data are for 2014–2016. In 2022, the University of Wisconsin's research generated comparable data for every county in the United States. The CDC is doing likewise for the years 2016–2019 at the municipal level and even at census tract scales. (See below and chapter 5 for discussions that show that the geographical patterns have not changed much).

Table 2.5 presents data on seven health-related metrics, standardized as best we could around the years 2014 to 2016. The first two metrics are critical because they are overall measures of self-reported health and age-adjusted death rates. We included five other health-related metrics: obesity, current smoker, binge drinking, vaccination for influenza, and asthma prevention. The data are sorted by broad categories of educational achievement, and race/ethnicity, and age. A major limitation of these data is that most are self-reported, and experience tells us that some people do not accurately report because they do not want potential problems noted.[20,21]

Beginning at the top of the table, the data show a clear difference by educational achievement. With the exception of binge drinking, college graduates have the highest self-declarations of good health, along with the lowest prevalence of obesity and smoking. With regard to race/ethnicity, note the extremely low rates and proportions of health risks among the state's Asian residents. New Jersey's Black residents have the highest death rates and the highest rates of obesity, smoking, and asthma. Hispanic respondents self-declared the lowest levels of overall health, and whites reported the highest levels of binge drinking. Please note that some of these estimates are based on small sample sizes and could be unstable.

County Comparisons

Information on health indicators for every county in the United States is readily available to the public.[6] We can report that New Jersey's age-adjusted death rate had been falling more rapidly than that for the nation as a whole. In 1990, the U.S. age-adjusted death rate was 938.0 per 100,000 population compared with the New Jersey rate of 949.9. A little more than a quarter century later, in 2016, the U.S. rate was 728.8 per 100,000 population, and New Jersey's had fallen to 669.1. In other words, before COVD-19, the state went from 1.2 percent higher to about 9 percent lower rate than that for the nation as a whole, a remarkable change.

There is no denying the intrastate variation in health outcomes and contributing factors in New Jersey. The impact of COVID-19 on the geography of NJ health is a focus of chapter 5.

In 2016, seven New Jersey counties had higher age-adjusted death rates than the U.S. rate: Atlantic, Camden, Cape May, Cumberland, Gloucester, Ocean, and Salem. All seven of these counties are located in the southern part of the state. Only one southern New Jersey county, Burlington, was not in this unenviable list. Also, in 2016 Essex and Passaic counties had the highest age-adjusted death rates outside of southern New Jersey.

Figure 2.1 clearly shows that the geography of health outcomes and health factors for New Jersey counties did not change as of 2020. The same seven southern counties ranked 19, 18, 17, 21, 15, 9, and 20, although Ocean County's outcomes did improve. Essex and Passaic ranked 16 and 14, respectively, in health outcomes in 2020.

Why is there so much variation within this state? Detailed data provided by the University of Wisconsin's County Health Rankings Reports point to persistent differences in health behaviors, clinical care, and social, economic, and environmental factors. But this prompts the question of why do these exist and persist? Although simple answers often are wrong, we provide two for consideration. First, the gap between wealth belt counties (Hunterdon, Morris, Bergen, and a portion of Somerset) and relatively poor ones (Cumberland, Salem, Atlantic, and Cape May) has grown and may be reflected in health factors. Second, modern society privileges education, which builds even more wealth and advantage.[23]

To examine our two simplistic answers, we correlated New Jersey county health outcomes and health risk factor rankings with three socioeconomic status metrics in 2019 (Table 2.6). We chose best public schools as a metric because the literature suggests that people with young families often dismiss living in places that do not have good public schools. Gasset[24] states, "When you buy a home, you are buying more than just the building, you are purchasing a lifestyle." In other words, high-quality schools are stronger predictors of a good lifestyle than are crime and safety, sidewalks and street lighting, highway accessibility, major conveniences, distance from railroad tracks, highway noise, walkability, access to trains, and nightlife. A second study[25] listed low

Table 2.6

Rank Correlations between Two Health Indicators and Three Socioeconomic Status Metrics, New Jersey Counties, 2020

Metric, Rank	Health Outcomes, 2020[6]	Health Factors, 2020[6]
Median household income, 2017[26]	0.87*	0.96*
Percentage of college graduates, 2017[26]	0.82*	0.83*
Best public schools, 2020[23]	0.78*	0.88*

* $P \leq 0.01$.
SOURCE: University of Wisconsin Population Health Institute. New Jersey 2020. County Health Rankings & Roadmaps,[6] Niche.com (2019).[23] and U.S. Census Bureau.[26]

noise as the most important metric for neighborhood quality, with good schools rated second. The best school metric was derived from measures of student test scores, graduation rates, ratings of teacher quality, and student and parent reviews.[23] We believe the best school metric represents a variety of the upstream indicators associated with health, such as access to health care, transportation options, retail services, and recreational opportunities.

Wealth does not tell the entire story of health outcome and behavior disparities. Yet the privileges associated with wealth are the place to start. Efforts to gain greater equity in opportunity are part of the story of every chapter of this book.

Historical Development of a Healthy New Jersey

The data and results of our analysis above require a discussion about other factors that connect to wealth and help account for New Jersey's health outcomes and the upstream predictors of health. In some ways, the expression "the apple doesn't fall far from the tree" characterizes the development of New Jersey. Even though the Revolutionary War was fought to disengage from the British Empire, the United States developed policies and practices, at least initially, that heavily borrowed from the British. In addition, New Jersey has been markedly influenced by its location "across the pond" and its situation between two of the largest cities in the United States. The next sections review the following New Jersey attributes and their health implications:

- Population movement (immigration and migration).
- Industrialization.
- Moderate climate and environment.
- Political moderation.

Immigration

As one of the original colonies, New Jersey has a history of welcoming those seeking a better life, particularly immigrants from Europe. Although Ellis Island is widely thought of as being in New York, it is located politically and geographically in New Jersey. Indeed, the 12 million immigrants who disembarked at Ellis Island actually began their new lives on the shores of this state.[27,28]

Immigration to the United States peaked in 1910 and declined during World War I. The current level of migration represents a second peak, albeit this remains heavily debated. Between 2000 and 2017, 580,000 foreign-born immigrants settled in New Jersey, which was the third-largest number of immigrants settling in the United States (after California and New York). As a result, New Jersey's foreign-born population is more than 20 percent.[29] The most common country of origin for recent immigrants to New Jersey is India, with many others from the People's Republic of China and South Korea. Ethnic Asian New Jersey residents had the lowest death rates and best indicators for every health-related indicator. Because most of these new immigrants have settled in the northern part of the state, the higher age-adjusted death rates for counties in southern New Jersey make sense.

Shaw explains that New Jersey appeals to immigrants because of the high degree of religious and political freedom and good economic opportunities that the state provides.[28] At an earlier time, these opportunities were associated with industrialization. Indeed, many of our early immigrants provided the labor for the state's industries to expand rapidly. During the period 1830 to 1880, immigrants from Ireland, Germany, and Great Britain filled the state's labor pool. After 1880, many immigrants came from Poland, Italy, Hungary, and Greece. In every national census since 1840, New Jersey has been one of the states with the highest proportion of foreign-born residents.[30] During the nineteenth century, these immigrants primarily settled in Essex, Hudson, and Passaic counties, and especially in the industrial cities of Newark, Jersey City, and Paterson. In 1956, Hungarians immigrated to New Jersey to flee the Hungarian revolution.

By the 1960s, immigrants from Puerto Rico and Cuba were eager to make New Jersey their home. Today, the immigration wave in New Jersey has become increasingly Asian.[31] While they have been extraordinarily successful in New Jersey, immigrants from many other countries have also succeeded in improving their status, including health behaviors, access to health care, and health outcomes. New Jersey is among the most diverse states by nationality, ethnicity and race, and factors associated with health outcomes.

Interstate Migration

New Jersey sits between two of the most dynamic cities in the United States. Many residents of New York City and Philadelphia moved to New Jersey for relief of that dynamism. For context, in 1790, the two most populated cities in the United States were New York City and Philadelphia with populations of 33,000 and 29,000, respectively. A half-century later, in 1840, New York City had a population of 313,000, Philadelphia had 94,000, and Brooklyn (which later became part of New York City) had an additional 36,000 residents. In New Jersey, Newark's population in 1840 was 17,300 and a small settlement was formed in Jersey City with a population of 3,100 people.[30]

The draw of New Jersey's less densely populated urban areas compared with those of New York City and Philadelphia provided opportune economic advantages, particularly in the early twentieth century when new major bridges and rail tunnels allowed people to commute across the Hudson and the Delaware Rivers. Between 1880 and 1930, the state's population grew from 1.1 million to 4 million. In that same year, Newark's population reached 442,000, and Jersey City's reached 316,000, the zenith for the population in both cities. Population growth was fueled by new immigrants as well as their second- and third-generation family members.[30] Simply put, immigrants played a dominant role in the growth of New Jersey's population, and this reality highly affected its health outcomes.

Industrialization

New Jersey began as a small agricultural colony of the British Empire, but it rapidly developed into a major industrial node, part of the U.S. manufacturing belt. The state turned out weapons during the Civil War, World War I, and World War II, and as well as many durable products between and after those wars. In 1960, New Jersey was one of only eight states that had more than 35 percent of their labor force working in manufacturing (Connecticut, Massachusetts, Michigan, New Hampshire, New Jersey, Ohio, Pennsylvania, and Rhode Island).[31] New Jersey's major ports in Newark, Elizabeth, and along the Delaware River made it an ideal location for manufacturing. The state's rail and highway networks reinforced water transportation.

The story of manufacturing in New Jersey is traced to the first secretary of the U.S. Treasury, Alexander Hamilton. Hamilton selected Paterson as the first major manufacturing center in the United States because of the seventy-seven-foot-high Great Falls located along the Passaic River, the resource providing the industrial power source of the age. Paterson manufactured silk, locomotives, pistols, and many other products, which attracted more Western European migrants and more industry. The Paterson Great Falls National Historical Park remains a major tourist attraction in the state today, and visitors can walk the Mill Mile to see the remnants of this great industrial past.[32]

For a good part of the twentieth century, New Jersey was the leading producer of chemicals in the United States. In fact, New Jersey was sometimes called "the nation's medicine chest" because it produced about 20 percent of all drugs manufactured in the United States.[31] In addition to drugs, the state produced organic and inorganic chemicals, with their manufacture concentrated in the northern and central part of the state in Essex, Middlesex, Passaic, Somerset, and Union counties. Part of the chemical manufacturing area was served by a rail line from the shores of the Arthur Kill to Perth Amboy, and the area was termed the "Chemical Coast."[33,34] Other clusters of chemical manufacturing existed in the cities of Trenton and Camden, as well as along the Delaware River in Gloucester and Salem counties.

Also during the twentieth century, New Jersey developed a motor vehicle manufacturing and assembly industry in Bergen, Mercer, Middlesex, and Union counties (in Mahwah, West Trenton, Edison, Edgewater, and Linden, respectively). These same areas produced books and other paper products as well as processed foods and other consumer products. For some time, the state had a robust electronic equipment–producing base. Space in New York City was in such demand that a good deal of the apparel industry moved across the river to New Jersey, particularly after rail and tunnel connections became available. Finally, petroleum-refining complexes appeared in Union and Middlesex Counties on the Arthur Kill and adjacent waterways, and in Paulsboro along the Delaware River in Gloucester County. The extensive reach of these facilities, visible along the Northeast Corridor rail line and the New Jersey Turnpike, often prompts outsiders to question how New Jersey can possibly be called the "Garden State."

Twentieth-century manufacturing in New Jersey concentrated in two places. The larger area was in the northeast, where Bergen, Essex, Hudson, Middlesex, Passaic, and Union counties tie their resources to the port of New York-New Jersey. The second concentration hugged the Delaware River in the cities of Camden and Trenton, as well as Camden, Gloucester, Mercer, Burlington, and Salem Counties. This concentration tied its resources to the Philadelphia metropolitan port complex.

In short, the Industrial Revolution stimulated high-density settlements in New Jersey and required the building of a sophisticated transportation infrastructure, including interconnected water, rail, and roads networks. New Jersey attracted immigrants and migrants and generated sufficient wealth to build impressive health care expertise and facilities across the state (see chapter 8). Yet we also know that industrialization led to severe contamination in many areas, especially in places near major industrial sites (see chapter 4). The legacy of this contamination became apparent as the industrial base declined and many locations closed. In 1969, the state had 894,000 manufacturing jobs; in 2015, the number was down to 238,000.[35]

The abandonment of many industrial sites opened up opportunities for new jobs in information, finance, and services, including health. Hudson County is a prominent example of this shift in the employment base. The county's population decreased between 1950 and 1960; Jersey City, the county's most prominent urban center, lost almost 8 percent of its population. Today, the population of Jersey City is rapidly rebounding. After the attack on the World Trade Center 2001, Jersey City became a relocation place for quite a few financial jobs. Simultaneously, the city has become one of the most ethnically diverse in the world, which is consistent with its location adjacent to Ellis Island.[36] The city's estimated 2018 population was 265,000 and growing until COVID-19 hit. The estimated population for 2022 fell to 257,000.

In many ways, Jersey City and Newark epitomize the perceptions of high-density living in New Jersey. Yet large portions of southern and northwestern New Jersey remain quite rural. Because of the legacy of home rule, the state's 565 municipal governments face challenges, including providing county and local health departments that struggle to meet the needs of their residents.

There is no denying the reality that the Industrial Revolution brought considerable wealth to New Jersey, but that wealth has not diffused across the state. It also brought a major environmental legacy discussed in chapter 4.

Mild Environment

New Jersey's ability to accommodate high-density urban and suburban development as well as maintain shore and mountain tourism and a strong agriculture base is possible because of the state's relatively mild and accommodating environment. The state as a whole has over fifty inches of rainfall annually. The southern part of the state has large supplies of groundwater, and large portions of the state have excellent fertile soils. These allow New

Jersey farmers to provide for not only the state's population, but also the appetites of its hungry neighbors (thus the Garden State label).

New Jersey has multiple climate regions. The relatively small northwestern climate zone is part of the Appalachian Highlands, characterized by colder winters and slopes that have hindered dense development elsewhere. Southern New Jersey is warmer and slightly drier than the northern and central parts of the state. It contains the Pine Barrens, a special ecological zone protected against suburban development. Without the Pine Barrens Commission, the area would now have a major airport and suburbs. The Atlantic coastal zone has moderate temperatures and winds compared with other shore areas in Florida, the Carolinas, and the northwest United States.[37] Nevertheless, tropical storms and nor'easters have battered the shoreline, causing some to reconsider the proper role of the shore as resort use rather than residential living.

The large central corridor of the state is the main pathway between New York City and Philadelphia, with a moderate climate and geology suitable for industrialization and urbanization. Furthermore, the state has small rivers and streams that with enhancements connect the Atlantic Ocean and the Delaware River. Large interstate roads now occupy areas adjacent to many of these rivers. New Jersey, in short, has a wide variety of geographical features in a small area. Yet the single most important detail is that the largest part of the state is made of coastal zone sediments, providing land that has been easy to develop.

Political Moderation

Without a doubt, the current political climate of New Jersey is also moderate. Facts demonstrate this political moderation:

- New Jersey is one of seven states with more registered Independent voters than are registered in either the Democratic or the Republican parties.
- Fully 77 percent of the registered voters in New Jersey are registered as either Independent or Democrat, a higher proportion than in forty-six other states.[38]

The current pattern of political moderation evolved over the second half of the twentieth century. After World War II, New Jersey leaned politically toward the Republican Party. Between 1948 and 1988, New Jersey voters picked Republican presidential candidates nine of eleven times. Since 1992, the Democratic presidential candidate was favored in all the presidential elections. Split gubernatorial races in New Jersey result in Democrats winning more often than Republicans. With the exception of the election of Chris Christie in 2010, Democrats have won all recent gubernatorial elections. The same pattern exists for senatorial elections with a relatively even split until the 1990s when Democratic Party candidates began to win in senatorial elections.

It is too simple to conclude that a Democratic plurality means that the state will embrace Health in All Policies (HiAP) and a culture of health, or that a Republican majority means that there is no chance for these efforts to succeed. As already noted, there are more registered Independent voters in the state than those registered for a political party. Thus, the ideas of HiAP and a culture of health must stand on their worth by convincing the vast majority of New Jersey voters they should be adopted.

It would be inaccurate to say that leading Republicans in New Jersey have not been moderate in their political leanings or they have not supported health. For example, former Republican Governor Tom Kean was chair of the Robert Wood Johnson Foundation, which contributed about $70 million to help establish the Cancer Institute of New Jersey, the New Jersey Nursing initiative, and the New Jersey Partnership for Healthy Kids. Under Governor Christine Todd Whitman's tenure, beach closings attributed to contamination and violations of the air quality standard or ozone markedly dropped. Governor Whitman also built a fund to buy and preserve open space and farmland in New Jersey. Her efforts at environmental protection led to her appointment as administrator of the U.S. Environmental Protection Agency (EPA) for several years.

Policy need not come solely from the governor and the state legislature. The well-known Mount Laurel affordable housing policy was enacted by the New Jersey Supreme Court with the goal of making every town responsible for providing at least some affordable housing.[39] In 1985, the New Jersey Supreme Court created the Abbott school district program to provide resources to thirty-one districts in the state that were found by the court to have inadequate financial resources so they could upgrade the quality of public school education[40] (see chapter 7).

These actions demonstrate the strong political and judicial support for both environmental health and public education in New Jersey. The state's population also supports health-related actions. For example, the Yale

University Program on Climate Change surveyed Americans to estimate their support for the contention that global warming is happening.[41] In the country as a whole, 70 percent agreed that climate change was occurring; in New Jersey, 74 percent of residents said it was (rank 5 among the states). Within the state, fifteen of New Jersey's twenty-one counties reported values higher than the national average. Four of the six reporting lower support were in southern New Jersey counties; the remaining two were in the northwest part of the state.[42]

As this discussion shows, New Jersey state government and the people as a whole are willing to press for tough policy changes. The large number of Independent voters means the state can offer new measures and practices that will improve public health. Should HiAP and a culture of health be presented to the public as worthwhile—a process for their collective benefit—they are more than likely to be adopted and move New Jersey along a healthier path.

References

1   Moore P. New Jersey: the least liked state in America. *YouGovAmerica*, July 1, 2015. https://today.yougov.com/topics/society/articles-reports/2015/07/01/new -jersey-least-liked-state-america

2   Legra J. Why New Jersey is the most hated state. *HuffPost Life*, August 6, 2015. https://www.huffpost.com/entry/why-new-jersey-is-the-most-hated-state_b _7951036

3   Monmouth University Polling Institute. Quality of life index stable; but desire to exit Jersey ticks up. April 25, 2022. https://www.monmouth.edu/polling-institute /reports/monmouthpoll_nj_042522/. Accessed September 22, 2022.

4   Quora. What are real people from New Jersey like? https://www.quora.com /What-are-real-people-from-New-Jersey-like. Accessed September 22, 2022.

5   Bernardo J. South Jersey secession: two views outsider sees a valid complaint. *New York Times*, October 18, 1981. https://www.nytimes.com/1981/10/18/nyregion /south-jersey-secession-two-views-outsider-sees-a-valid-complaint.html

6   University of Wisconsin Population Health Institute. New Jersey 2020. County Health Rankings & Roadmaps. https://www.countyhealthrankings.org/app /new-jersey/2020/overview

7   New Jersey rankings and facts. *U.S. News & World Report*, 2019. https://www .usnews.com/news/best-states/new-jerseyNews Best States.

8   Witters D. Hawaii tops U.S. in wellbeing for record 7th time. Gallup News, February 27, 2019. https://news.gallup.com/poll/247034/hawaii-tops-wellbeing -record-7th-time.aspx

9   Happiest States 2019. World Population Review. https://worldpopulationreview .com/state-rankings/happiest-states

10 Hall B, Kerr ML. *1991–1992 Green Index: A State-by-State Guide to the Nation's Environmental Health*. Washington, DC: Island Press; 1991.

11 Bernardo R. 2017's Happiest states in America. *WalletHub*, September 11, 2017. https://web.archive.org/web/20171224074156/https://wallethub.com/edu/happiest-states/6959/

12 Porter D. 1st COVID-19 death in New Jersey was veteran horseman. *AP News*, March 11, 2020. https://apnews.com/article/8ae6fdfa2fdf6c87ab6608e109453b51

13 Communicable Disease Service, NJ Department of Health. New Jersey COVID-19 Dashboard. Accessed April 29, 2021. https://www.nj.gov/health/cd/topics/covid2019_dashboard.shtml

14 Symons M. COVID-19 drives NJ's death rate to highest level in 75 years. *NJ101.5*, March 9, 2021. https://nj1015.com/covid-19-drives-njs-death-rate-to-highest-level-in-75-years/

15 Yates R. How many N.J. lives has COVID-19 taken? More than you've been told. Here's why. *NJ.com*, October 25, 2020. https://www.nj.com/coronavirus/2020/10/how-many-nj-lives-has-covid-19-taken-more-than-youve-been-told-heres-why.html

16 Fallon S. Coronavirus NJ: a timeline of events from first cases to first casualties. NorthJersey.com, March 10, 2020 https://www.northjersey.com/story/news/health/2020/03/10/coronavirus-new-jersey-timeline-events-covid-covid-19/4964918002/

17 Rosenthal BM. Density is New York City's big "enemy" in the coronavirus fight. *New York Times*, March 23, 2020. https://www.nytimes.com/2020/03/23/nyregion/coronavirus-nyc-crowds-density.html

18 Centers for Medicare & Medicaid Services. CMS announces new measures to protect nursing home residents from COVID-19 [press release]. CMS.gov *Newsroom*, March 13, 2020. https://www.cms.gov/newsroom/press-releases/cms-announces-new-measures-protect-nursing-home-residents-covid-19

19 Centers for Disease Control and Prevention. Considerations for retirement communities and independent living facilities. Updated August 24, 2021. https://www.cdc.gov/coronavirus/2019-ncov/community/retirement/considerations.html

20 Brener ND, Kann L, Kinchen SA, et al. Methodology of the youth risk behavior surveillance system. *MMWR Recomm Rep*. 2004;53(RR-12):1–13. https://www.cdc.gov/mmwr/preview/mmwrhtml/rr5312a1.htm

21 Weinstein ND, Nicolich M. Correct and incorrect interpretations of correlations between risk perceptions and risk behaviors. *Health Psychol*. 1993;12(3):235–245. doi:10.1037//0278-6133.12.3.235

22 Center for Health Statistics and Informatics, New Jersey State Health Assessment Data (NJSHAD), New Jersey Department of Health. https://www.nj.gov/health/chs/

23 2019 New Jersey counties with the best public schools. Niche.com. https://www.niche.com/places-to-live/search/counties-with-the-best-public-schools/s/new-jersey/

24 Gassett B. What to look for when searching for a neighborhood. Maximum Exposure Real Estate, January 19, 2015. https://www.maxrealestateexposure.com/what-to-look-for-when-searching-for-a-neighborhood/

25 11 Smart things to look for in a new neighborhood. *Mental Floss*, May 3, 2016. https://www.mentalfloss.com/article/78765/11-smart-things-look-new -neighborhood

26 U.S. Census Bureau. Decennial census of population and housing tables 2010. https://www.census.gov/programs-surveys/decennial-census/data/tables.2010 .List_1115666347.html

27 Gibson CJ, Lennon E. Historical census statistics on the foreign-born population of the United States: 1850 to 1990. U.S. Census Bureau Working Paper POP-WP029. February 1999. https://www.census.gov/library/working-papers/1999 /demo/POP-twps0029.html

28 Shaw DV. *Immigration and Ethnicity in New Jersey History.* Trenton, NJ: New Jersey Historical Commission, Department of State; 1994. http://hdl.handle.net /10929/24561

29 Zong J, Batalova J, Burrows M. Frequently requested statistics on immigrants and immigration in the United States. Migration Policy Institute *Spotlight*, March 17, 2022. https://www.migrationpolicy.org/article/frequently-requested-statistics -immigrants-and-immigration-united-states

30 U.S. Census Bureau. *Historical Statistics of the United States, Colonial Times to 1970.* 2 vols. Washington, DC: U.S. Government Printing Office; 1975. https:// fraser.stlouisfed.org/title/historical-statistics-united-states-237

31 States with the most immigrants. Lattice Publishing, July 2, 2018. https://www .latticepublishing.com/blog/states-with-the-most-immigrants

32 Paterson Great Falls National Historical Park, New Jersey. U.S. National Park Service. https://www.nps.gov/pagr/index.htm

33 Chemical Coast. Wikipedia, updated May 1, 2022. https://en.wikipedia.org/wiki /Chemical_Coast

34 Larrabee RM. The Port of New York & New Jersey: a leading indicator of globalization. PowerPoint Presentation. March 2006. Paper presented at: Transportation Research Forum, 47th Annual Transportation Research Forum; March 23–25, 2006; New York, NY. https://ageconsearch.umn.edu/record/208050

35 Greenberg MR. *Siting Noxious Facilities: Integrating Location Economics and Risk Analysis to Protect Environmental Health and Investments.* New York: Routledge; 2018.

36 Zeitlinger R. This New Jersey city is the most diverse in the nation—again. *NJ.com*, February 13, 2018. https://www.nj.com/hudson/2018/02/jersey_city_retains_title _as_most_diverse_city_in.html

37 Office of the New Jersey State Climatologist. New Jersey climate overview. Rutgers University; n.d. https://climate.rutgers.edu/stateclim/?target=NJCoverview

38 Cook R. Registering by party: where the Democrats and Republicans are ahead. *Sabato's Crystal Ball*, July 12, 2018. https://centerforpolitics.org/crystalball/articles /registering-by-party-where-the-democrats-and-republicans-are-ahead/

39 Massey DS, Albright L, Casciano R, et al. *Climbing Mount Laurel: The Struggle for Affordable Housing and Social Mobility in an American Suburb.* Princeton, NJ: Princeton University Press; 2013.

40 Ford A. Looking back and towards the future: Abbott Preschool after 20 years. *New America*, May 8, 2018. https://www.newamerica.org/education-policy /edcentral/looking-back-and-towards-future-abbott-preschool-after-20-years/

41   Deeg K, Lyon E, Leiserowitz A, et al. Who is changing their mind about global warming and why? Yale Program on Climate Change Communication *Climate Note*, January 9, 2019. https://climatecommunication.yale.edu/publications/who -is-changing-their-mind-about-global-warming-and-why/

42   Greenberg MR. Is public support for environmental protection decreasing? An analysis of U.S. and New Jersey data. *Environ Health Perspect.* 2004;112(2):121–125. doi:10.1289/ehp.6648

3

Transportation Drives Population Shifts

———————————————————●

"On the New Jersey Turnpike, no one
can hear you scream."
—Richard Pryor, 1988[1]

Richard Pryor's unheard scream is not what Alfred Driscoll anticipated
when he became governor of New Jersey in 1946. New Jersey and United
States as a whole experienced euphoria from winning World War II, and the
nation was gearing up to switch from manufacturing war goods to consumer
products. Optimism prevailed, and the fertility rate jumped from 2.28 children
per woman during the war years to 3.32 after the war's end, thus creating a baby
boom. The U.S. gross national product increased two and a half times after the
war, nothing short of an amazing demonstration of nation's economic and
political prowess.[2,3] This chapter has four objectives:

1 Review major highway systems built to facilitate automobile and
  suburban-oriented lifestyles.
2 Discuss the consequences of highway building, housing, deindustrialization, and other policy decisions that increased suburban sprawl
  and hastened the decline of older cities.

3 Review the health-related consequences of these actions.
4 Consider the response of government, not-for-profit and private
   organizations, and the public to these health-related consequences.

Highways Have Health Consequences

The Republican governor and his New Jersey constituents faced a daunting
transportation problem. Automobile sales increased rapidly after the war,
and the state's roads, many built during the 1920s (e.g., Routes 1, 3, 9, 17, 18,
21, 22, 27, 46, 130, and others), could not accommodate the growing volume
of vehicular traffic. Frustrated people and businesses complained of traffic
congestion. Furthermore, having just fought for freedom on the world stage,
it seemed un-American to keep an increasingly affluent population in small
apartments in urban centers. Rather than constrain people and businesses,
especially in the aging cities of the Northeast and Midwest, the population
wanted automobiles so they could tour the country, travel to work in style,
buy a bigger house, and expand their businesses to new locations.

Unlike Europe, the war did not devastate the United States, so the nation
could afford to invest in a highway expansion program. The German auto-
bahns were an appealing illustration of what was possible in a densely settled
state such as New Jersey.[4] Indeed, Hitler's limited access, high-speed highways were extremely popular with the German public, a fact noted by General Eisenhower, an expert in logistics, as he directed the invasion of Europe.

The Turnpike

As the most densely populated state, New Jersey arguably needed a major
highway program more than other states did. Governor Driscoll's signature
solution was the New Jersey Turnpike, a 118-mile toll road connecting the
George Washington Bridge at the northern end to the Delaware Memorial
Bridge at the southern. The idea of the Turnpike was appealing:

- The highway would have no traffic lights or stop signs; it would have
  clearly demarcated exits that would intersect with state and local roads.
- New Jersey taxpayers would not directly pay for the highway; toll
  booths would collect tolls from users, including many from out
  of state.

- The highway would have its own police and service vehicles, with rest stops providing opportunities for gas, food, and restrooms so that travelers would not have to exit for these services.

The New Jersey state legislature created the New Jersey Turnpike Authority (NJTA) in 1949 as a no-frills entity. The agency had the powers necessary to build and operate the road, including bonding to pay for expansion. The process involved clearing factories, a railroad yard, and farms to provide the Turnpike with straight runs. One clear run goes directly through a massive petroleum refinery and a series of tank farms in Elizabeth, New Jersey, a run that surely blemished (and continues to blemish) the state's image. However, during the late 1940s and early 1950s, utility trumped aesthetics. The Turnpike was so bare bones that the NJTA dealt with heavy air pollution days by simply hanging speed signs on the road and having state troopers guide drivers through the fog.[5]

It would be unfair to conclude that Governor Driscoll and others who advocated so strongly for the Turnpike had no sense of design. Capturing public expectations in his fourth annual message to the legislature in 1951, Alfred Driscoll stated, "Modern highways are a prime wartime requirement. We will be constantly examining our highway program in light of changing circumstances. We expect the Turnpike to be completed this year.... We may confidently expect the Turnpike, upon its completion, to be one of the nation's greatest wartime and peacetime assets" (13).[6]

The issues that challenged building the Turnpike included private efforts to buy parts of the right of way and resell the parcels to the NJTA at a profit; the need to move people, businesses, and farmers; and the reality that the Turnpike bypassed many communities, undermining their economies. On the positive side, the Turnpike was a major feat of engineering for its time. The highway opened on November 30, 1951, for traffic between the Delaware Memorial Bridge (interchange 1) and Woodbridge, New Jersey (exit 10). At the opening, Governor Driscoll stated, "The Turnpike has permitted New Jersey to emerge from behind the billboards, the hot dog stands and the junkyards. Motorists can now see the beauty of the real New Jersey."[7]

We would certainly not designate the entirety of the Turnpike as a road to view the beauty of New Jersey. On the other hand, it is a relatively safe road per driven mile.[8] By way of comparison, New York's 105-mile Taconic Parkway (running from Westchester County northward to Interstate 90) looks like a golf course along much of its winding pathway. The Taconic is also the deadliest road in the state of New York. It suffers from narrow, two-lane construction that many drivers find difficult to navigate, with many drivers causing accidents because of speeding and ending up on the wrong side of the road.[9]

Words cannot do justice to the Turnpike. It needs to be experienced. To feel the experience of a Turnpike traveler when the highway first opened, we encourage viewing the twenty-three-minute newsreel "New Jersey Turnpike Super Highway 1950s" on YouTube. The film characterizes the Turnpike as "the most modern, the most heavily traveled highway in the world—triumph of engineering skill and far-sighted planning! Driving on the New Jersey Turnpike is like entering a new world; a world without stoplights or sharp curves; a world created for motoring pleasure."[5]

The Turnpike newsreel idealized the desirability of auto ownership and the freedom it offered. In one clip, New Jersey state troopers drive up to a stopped vehicle and exhibit remarkable patience while assisting a motorist. In another clip, a service truck operator demonstrates superhuman care and patience while replacing a fan belt. Best of all, an attractive "pikette" emerges from a Turnpike service station to give a set of maps to a man driving to Florida. All three of these highlights occurred in traffic resembling that of a lightly traveled, four-lane suburban road.

The black-and-white images and verbal messages of the newsreel were consistent with those of the popular 1950s television show *Leave It to Beaver*. The Cleaver family lived on Pine Street in a fictitious suburb named Mayfield. Beaver, a preteen played by Jerry Mathers, had a traditional suburban family. His dad, Ward, dressed in a suit and tie as he drove his car to a white-collar job. Beaver's mother, June, also was always perfectly dressed. His teenage brother, Wally, was a three-sport athlete who proudly wore his letter jacket enhanced with a big "M" for Mayfield. In other words, the show idealized the image of the suburbs and automobile ownership. When suburban families traveled in their shiny new cars, they could experience the Turnpike—stopping at the rest stops and purchasing Turnpike and other New Jersey memorabilia. Figure 3.1 is an example of vintage postcards that travelers could purchase at one of the Turnpike rest stops during the 1950s.[10]

Rutgers professors Michael Rockland and Angus Gillespie's book *Looking for America on the New Jersey Turnpike* offers a marvelous characterization of the Turnpike, covering both the utility of the road and the spirit it represents: "cold, dark, austere, a largely lifeless environment over which

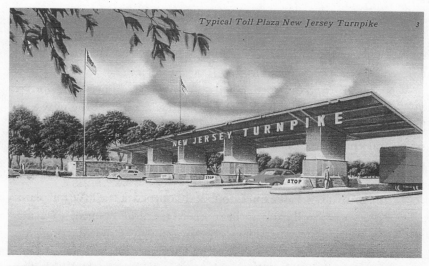

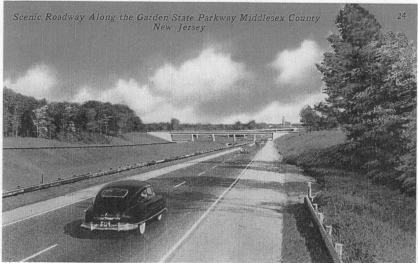

FIGURE 3.1 1950s postcards from the New Jersey Turnpike. (*Source:* New Jersey Historical Society.)

humans scamper as fast as their motor vehicles, and the law, will allow. It's like a legacy from the 1950s and the World of Tomorrow. It is ugly. But it's also a symbol of something that's very American."[11]

Currently, the Turnpike has twenty-nine interchanges, beginning with the Delaware Memorial Bridge at milepost 1.2 in the south and ending with a connector to the George Washington Bridge in the north. From

Mansfield Township (exit 6) and northward, the Turnpike has twelve lanes (six northbound and six southbound). The outer lanes are open to cars and trucks, whereas the inner lanes are limited to cars. The Turnpike also has twelve service plazas named for New Jersey luminaries.[12]

When the Turnpike opened, it had only four lanes. However, traffic was so substantial that by 1955 the NJTA proposed widening the highway to six lanes between exit 4 (Mount Laurel) and exit 10 (Woodbridge). Additional structural changes to the Turnpike helped improved traffic flow. Some twenty-first century improvements include

- 2004. Two E-Z Pass express tollbooths opened at the I8W toll plaza.
- 2004. A new toll plaza at the southern terminus opened, featuring a gateway lighthouse and walkway over fourteen southbound lanes, five northbound lanes and two E-Z Pass lanes.
- 2005. A new exit (15W) opened, providing access to the Frank Lautenberg rail station (Secaucus) where trains from Bergen County connect to the Amtrak rail line.
- 2011. All toll plazas began accepting E-Z Pass.
- 2009–2014. A major widening project between exits 6 an 9 included a restructured exit 8 in East Windsor. The project also improved interchanges and continued the northern Turnpike pattern of four sets of three lanes each.[13]

Shipkowski reported that the 2009 to 2014 Turnpike expansion project was one of the largest road construction projects in North America.[14] Colimore reported that the expansion led many drivers to sing the Turnpike's praises.[15] The NJTA reported a 3.5 percent increase in traffic in 2016, the fifth straight year of increased traffic and toll collection revenue due to the expansion.[16]

Drivers have complained about tolls and congestion on the Turnpike almost since it opened in 1951. Davis noted that at least part of the resentment about the tolls stems from the fact that had the Federal-Aid Highway Act of 1956 funded the Turnpike it would have been a freeway, receiving 80 percent or more of its costs from the federal government.[17] Because the state built the highway before Congress passed the act, it continues to collect tolls—a nagging thorn in the side of the state's commuters.

Despite Turnpike widening, New Jersey commuters still struggle with congestion. The worst congestion is on the Lincoln Tunnel connection between New Jersey and New York City, followed by the connection to the George Washington Bridge. Next in congestion are the connections to Routes 1 and 9 in Newark and the Pulaski Skyway to Jersey City. Although commuters complain about these backups, those who have traveled by auto in and around Los Angeles might feel right at home. Martucci identified fourteen U.S. cities with the worst traffic congestion and longest commutes in the nation.[18] New York City ranked number one, but Jersey City ranked second, and Newark ranked fourth. Three of the remaining cities in the list were in California. Indeed, Higgs reports that ten of the twenty-five worst traffic hotspots across the nation are in the Los Angeles area.[19]

Many truck drivers deliberately avoid the Turnpike and its tolls, and they routinely complain about traffic congestion and accidents along New Jersey roadways. Salant has reported that operating costs for truckers are highest in Texas, with New Jersey ranking second.[20] On the other hand, the traffic congestion causing problems for some truckers is a benefit for others. In October 2018, Quinn and Breeze[21] reported that 61 million people lived within 250 miles of the New Jersey Turnpike—in other words, the Turnpike serves the largest residential population in the entire United States. As they wrote, "No other market in the country has the ability to reach as many people with same-day delivery as this one."

The Interstate Highway System

President Eisenhower took notice of the success of the New Jersey and Pennsylvania turnpikes and advocated for an extensive federal highway system. General revenues would fund building the system, and gasoline taxes would then support it. Fishman noted that the building of nation's interstate highway network was the largest public works program since the pyramids.[22]

While the Turnpike forms the heart and probably the soul of New Jersey's highway system, the federal highway system keeps it all moving. The state currently has all or parts of eight federal interstate highways within its boundaries[23] (Table 3.1). Interstate 80 (I-80) is the second longest interstate in the nation. Almost sixty-nine miles of its 2,899 miles are in New Jersey. Originally called Christopher Columbus Highway, I-80 begins at the George Washington Bridge, runs across the northern part of the state to the Delaware Water Gap, and continues to its western terminus in San Francisco. Glass reports that I-80 is the ninth most dangerous highway in

Table 3.1
Interstate Highways in New Jersey

Interstate Number	Length, Miles	Eastern or Northern Terminus	Western or Southern Terminus	Construction Began
I-76	3.08	I-295/Route 42 in Bellmawr	I-76 in Camden	1964
I-78	67.83	Holland Tunnel in Jersey City	Toll bridge at the Delaware River in Phillipsburg	1957
I-80	68.54	I-95 in Teaneck	Toll bridge at the Delaware Water Gap in Hardwick Township	1956
I-95	88.99	George Washington Bridge in Fort Lee	Toll bridge at the Delaware River in Florence Township	1956
I-195	34.17	Garden State Parkway and Route 34 in Wall Township	Route 20 in Hamilton Township	1968
I-278	2.00	Goethals Bridge in Elizabeth	US 1 and 9 in Linden	1961
I-280	17.85	NJ Turnpike in Kearney	I-80 in Parsippany-Troy Hills	1958
I-287	67.54	Route 17 in Mahwah	NJ Turnpike in Edison	1961
I-295	76.56	Toll bridge at Scudder Falls in Ewing	US 40 in Pennsville Township	1958
I-495	3.45	Lincoln Tunnel in Weehawken	New Jersey Turnpike in Secaucus	1961
I-676	4.75	U.S. 30 at the Ben Franklin Bridge in Camden	I-76 in Gloucester City	1964

SOURCE: New Jersey Department of Transportation.[23,25]

the United States, with never-ending semitrucks moving at high speeds, in sections with dangerous winds and insufficient bridges, particularly through the Midwest. I-80 accounted for 209 highway fatalities in 2019 alone (7.21 fatalities per 100 miles of road).[24]

The Lure of the Suburbs

The 1956 Federal-Aid (Interstate) Highway Act guided American land use in ways not planned or anticipated. For example, the highway system was supposed to help Northeast and Midwest cities by easing traffic congestion and improving intercity transportation. Instead, some interstate highways cut through cities, destroying neighborhoods. New beltways around cities allowed drivers to avoid the central business district (CBD) altogether, reducing the traffic required for robust commerce. New businesses and suburban shopping malls popped up like mushrooms around the new beltways and interchanges, providing access to amenities required for those rushing home to or between the suburbs.[26]

Creation of the highway system was not a small influence on urban America. In 1999, the Fannie May Foundation sponsored a survey to rank the most important influences that shaped metropolitan America from 1950 to the end of the century.[22] The top ten influences were

1 The 1956 Interstate Highway Act and increasing importance of the automobile.
2 The Federal Housing Administration mortgage financing program and accompanying subdivision regulations.
3 The massive industrial decline of central cities.
4 Urban renewal, most notably downtown clearing, redevelopment, and public housing projects as part of the 1949 Housing Act.
5 Mass-produced suburban tract homes, epitomized by Levittown, NY (built 1947–1951); Levittown, PA (built 1952–1958); and Willingboro Township, NJ (started in 1958).
6 Housing segregation and job discrimination.
7 Enclosed shopping malls.
8 Sunbelt-style sprawl.
9 Air conditioning.
10 Urban unrest during the 1960s.

Fishman[22] emphasizes the power of the federal government to both intentionally and unintentionally reshape the American metropolis, spurring suburban growth and undermining central cities and their older industrial hinterlands. More than a half century after this pattern emerged, it is still visible.

Mortgage and Subdivision Policies

Veterans returning from war need jobs and other benefits. After World War II, those benefits for U.S. veterans included access to education and a mortgage program originally devised during the New Deal to stimulate a weak economy. Before the Federal Housing Administration (FHA) program in 1949, potential homebuyers typically had to put down half of the cost of a house and pay high mortgage interest rates, often for decades. The FHA program markedly lowered both requirements. For example, 44 percent of Americans were homeowners in 1940. By 1970, the proportion was 63 percent; in 2000 it reached 66 percent.[27] However, the FHA program did not provide similar benefits for homes in city neighborhoods. This policy, along with accompanying subdivision regulations, made suburban access for Black Americans and other poor populations difficult.

Suburban Housing Developments

Innovations in premanufactured housing by Abraham Levitt and his sons, and the changes in FHA financing, allowed many Americans to achieve suburban homeownership. The goal of a white picket fence, green lawn, modern appliances, and an automobile filled their dreams. Tens of thousands of new homes sprang up to fulfill those dreams, with most new homes located on inexpensive land near newly constructed highways. Rosenberg has noted how Levittowns epitomized the postwar, middle-class housing boom.[28] In 1946, groundbreaking on 4,000 acres of potato fields in Hempstead, Long Island, began the building of America's largest housing development. The massive development, designated Levittown, New York, was complete in 1951. A second massive development sprang up in Levittown, Pennsylvania (1952–1958), and a third emerged in Willingboro Township, New Jersey (1952–1958). The growth of Levittowns and other massive suburban subdivisions markedly changed the American landscape, particularly in the Northeast and Midwest.[29]

Keeping with 1950s television examples, we offer *The Honeymooners*. Its star, Ralph Kramden, played by Jackie Gleason, drove a bus on New York's Madison Avenue. The Kramdens had a tiny apartment with one window in the kitchen and an icebox (not a refrigerator), the epitome of white poverty in urban America. Conversely, the 1956 season of *I Love Lucy* begins with Lucy Ricardo, played by Lucille Ball, trying to convince her middle-class husband Ricky (Desi Arnaz) to leave Manhattan and move to a house in Connecticut—which they eventually do. These shows reinforced the 1950s views of urban life as less than ideal compared with the promise of the suburbs.

Sunbelt, Air Conditioning, and Enclosed Shopping Malls

Northeast and Midwest suburbs were not the only places that experienced accelerated growth after the war. The South and Southwest also experienced massive in-migration. The Sunbelt appealed to those who wanted to experience longer summers, shorter winters, and the feeling of open space. New roads, technical innovations, and land use policies disproportionately enhanced the attractiveness of both suburbs and the Sunbelt. Air conditioning became generally available in the 1950s, which had a marked impact on the growth of cities such as Las Vegas, Phoenix, and other cities that had previously been inhospitable because of their extreme heat and low rainfall.[30] By 2019, California, Texas, and Florida ranked number 1, 2, and 3 in population size, respectively, a status made possible by controlling indoor environments. Sunbelt attractiveness has not waned: the area recently experiencing the most population growth in the United States remains the triangular area bordered by Dallas–Fort Worth, Houston–Galveston, and San Antonio, Texas.[31]

Outdoor suburban malls first appeared in the 1950s. Located near the major new highways to draw in customers who had moved to the suburbs, these malls offered parking, at least two large department stores, and other amenities. As the new shopping centers spread, they became climate controlled, and they were designed and managed by national franchises. The malls drew retailing and wholesaling to the suburbs as well as parts of the financial industry.[32] They undermined both older CBDs and the shopping along the roads leading to them. Like the CBDs that had begun to decline in the 1950s, the suburban malls in the twenty-first century face increasing completion, particularly from online retailing and big-box stores.[33] As a result, many smaller malls have become "grayfields," defined by their massive, empty parking lots. The rapidly changing postpandemic economy has further contributed to this decline.

Manufacturing Decline

Northern cities and older industrial suburbs began to lose their competitive advantage for manufacturing during the 1950s. They had rail and water access, water and sewer service,[34] but they could not compete with suburban locations that had cheap, flat land that accommodated new production processes. The latter were enhanced by tax benefits and quick access to new federal highways. Slowly, industry moved to the suburbs, then to the Sunbelt, and then crossed the oceans to Asia, Europe, and Latin America in search of cheap, non-union labor and large tax benefits. Detroit, Buffalo, Philadelphia, Milwaukee, St. Louis, and the New Jersey cities of Newark, Jersey City, Paterson, Camden, Perth Amboy, and others became underfunded "Rust Belt" cities. Those left behind—essentially those marooned in declining urban places—had little opportunity, and the process increased the racial and income segregation that would erupt in the 1960s (see chapter 5).[34]

Urban Renewal

Even as the suburbs were becoming more appealing and affordable, some older city CBDs and their neighborhoods faced demolition as part of the Housing Act of 1949. The federal government worked with local governments to rebuild CBDs. This meant destroying parts of some downtowns and turning those locations into highways, parking lots, and new stores that did not prove appealing to consumers. The stated goal was to create a "suitable living environment," but the model for new housing, adapted from the British experience, was the monolithic high-rise apartment complexes. These structures were dark and had insufficient ventilation; the electricity routinely failed, and maintenance was a problem.[35] Many have since been replaced by less daunting structures.

Mieszkowski and Mills[36] calculated that, in 1950, 57 percent of residents lived in central cities, and 70 percent of jobs were located in them. By 1970, these numbers had decreased to 43 percent and 55 percent, respectively. Kopecy and Suen[37] examined the factors contributing to the decrease of population density from central cities to the suburbs between 1910 and 1970, and they concluded that rising incomes and the automobile were the major drivers. Furthermore, after 1950 the new highways expanded the reach of the automobile and substantially decreased the public's commuting time, loosening their commitment to cities.

Baum-Snow[38] makes a persuasive case for the role of highways in explaining post–World War II suburbanization, estimating that the new interstates passing through CBDs reduced the populations of forty-one center cities by 18 percent. New highways to the suburbs also facilitated white flight, especially after significant periods of unrest[39–41] (see chapters 5 and 6).

Health Consequences for Declining Cities

For some, movement to the suburbs or the Sunbelt resulted in a better quality of life. They found more personal and family space, access to large tracts of land with beautiful vistas, well-funded schools and public services, a more relaxed feeling, and more. All of these promote better health. For those who could not move, the result was disappointing: they remained stranded in declining cities with few resources or the public services needed to support them. There is a large literature on the relationship between sprawl and health.[42-60] Table 3.2 summarizes key observations from this literature.

Our original intent was to present a New Jersey case study at this point; however, readers may be more familiar with the experience of the Cross Bronx Expressway (CBE) cutting through neighborhoods in New York City. Robert Caro's Pulitzer Prize–winning biography of Robert Moses[61] focuses on the use of power to control land use in New York City, including building the CBE. That roadway specifically benefited suburban commuters between New Jersey, Queens, other parts of Long Island, Westchester County, and New England—but not the residents of the Bronx. Caro's book emphasizes the inequity of deliberately choosing to build the CBE through this area when other less impactful options were available.

For example, one of the authors of this book, Michael Greenberg, lived his early years on 169th Street in the Bronx, a short distance away from the path followed by the CBE as it went under the Grand Concourse at 174th Street. When the crews started dynamiting the hard rock to begin CBE construction, young boys (including myself) were completely captivated by what seemed like a World War II battle in their own neighborhood. This was great fun for boys, but many workers and business owners near the pathway for the new highway were irate when their offices experienced the vibrations from the explosions and rock removal. What the boys also did not know was east of where they lived, more than 1,500 families and businesses were removed for construction of the CBE (Figure 3.2). As a result, that area became one of the poorest in New York City, with limited opportunities for jobs and investment compared with other nearby neighborhoods.

More than a half century later, Kim et al.[62] proposed building decks over the CBE. Rather than focus on the moral argument for addressing the expressway's impact, they conducted cost-effectiveness analyses of building

Table 3.2
Health Consequences of Sprawl and Urban Decline

Health Consequence	Causes
Vehicle crashes; driver, passenger, and pedestrian injuries and deaths	• By 1960, more vehicle miles, often associated with substance abuse and distracted driving, result in about 50,000 deaths per year. • Safer cars, seatbelts, and roads reduce auto fatalities but do not increase pedestrian safety (especially when crossing high-speed roads with multiple lanes, no traffic lights, and no pedestrian overpasses or underpasses).
Air pollution	• More vehicle miles driven creates air pollution and contributes to increases in respiratory symptoms and greenhouse gases (see chapter 4).
Sedentary lifestyles	• Isolated streets and communities without good public transportation encourage driving rather than walking. • Sedentary living increases the probability of obesity, cardiovascular and cerebrovascular diseases, diabetes, and certain cancers. • Sedentary living decreases the ability to build relationships with friends and neighbors and to contribute social capital to community groups.
Loss of water quality and quantity	• More impervious surfaces result in the loss of forests and other green cover that slow the flow of contaminated material into surface water bodies and allow infiltration into groundwater sources.
Urban heat islands	• Cement, asphalt, and other dark surfaces lead to substantial increases in local temperatures, especially in areas without shade trees to absorb excess heat. • Lethal heat wave events occur in Chicago, Milwaukee, New York, and other metropolitan areas. • People with pre-existing health conditions, especially the poor, elderly, disabled, or those living by themselves without air-conditioning are at elevated risk for heat deaths.
Mental and physical health stress	• Automobile commuting can be physically and mentally stressful, particularly when there are long delays due to accidents, road construction, or bad weather conditions. • Some drivers suffer back strain or repetitive injuries, some may fall asleep at the wheel, and a few may respond to frustrating situations with road rage.
Environmental justice	• Noxious facilities are disproportionately located near areas occupied by the poor, ethnic/racial minorities, seniors, and disabled individuals. • New highways cutting through cities are disproportionately located near areas occupied by the poor, ethnic/racial minorities, seniors, and disabled individuals. • Exposure to these facilities increases physical and mental stress with health implications.

SOURCES: Baum-Snow (2007)[38]; Boustan (2010)[39]; Frey (1979)[40]; Ravitch (1978)[41]; Cockerham (2007)[43]; Berrigan and Troiano (2002)[44]; Semenza et al. (1996)[45]; Rathbone (1999)[46]; Kaplan et al. (1996)[47]; Wilson (2012)[48]; Newman and Kenworthy (1999)[49]; Wing (1993)[50]; Whitman et al. (1997)[51]; McCann and DeLille (2000)[52]; Dannenberg et al. (2011)[53]; Duany et al. (2000)[54]; National Research Council (1988)[55]; Pope et al. (1995)[56], CDC (1999)[57]; Thompson et al. (2003)[58]; CDC (1996)[59]; Frank (2000)[60].

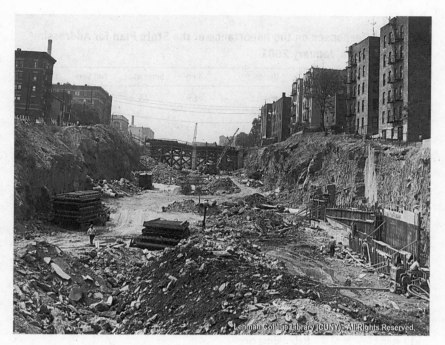

FIGURE 3.2 Construction of the Cross Bronx Expressway in 1962 cutting through the community and contributing to its decline. (*Source:* Lehman College Library (CUNY).)

a deck with parks. They estimated the health benefits from exercise, less air and noise pollution, a public area to relax and build social capital, reduce stress, and reclaim some of the reduced property values. Citing several other projects in Seattle and Boston, and noting the use of this approach in Europe, their study focused only on residents who live within a half-mile from the proposed decks. The authors offered their proposal as a "low-cost public works project for a low income community (380)."[62] The project likely would benefit community health in poor and underserved areas.

Public Concerns about Traffic Congestion and Sprawl

New Jersey residents lived with dense traffic and sprawl for generations. Have they simply accepted these conditions as intractable? An excellent opportunity to assess the public's perception of the traffic congestion issue occurred in 2001 when residents were asked to rate the importance of five issues included in the newly developed state plan. Table 3.3

Table 3.3

Percent of Responses on the Importance of the State Plan for Addressing Public Concerns, January 2001

Question	Option	Very	Somewhat	Not Very	Don't Know
How important is the following as part of the NJ state plan? (n = 408)	Easing traffic congestion	69	25	6	1
	Stopping suburban sprawl	44	42	10	4
	Rebuilding city centers	58	32	8	2
	Preserving open space	63	27	9	1
	Providing economic growth	69	27	3	1

Question	Option	A lot	Some	A little	No progress
Progress in your community in reaching each goal over the last 10 years? (n = 395)	Easing traffic congestion	5	19	33	40
	Stopping suburban sprawl	8	18	33	28
	Rebuilding city centers	14	28	32	17
	Preserving open space	21	34	26	14
	Providing economic growth	23	40	6	6

SOURCE: Eagleton Poll archive.[56]

shows that the public identified the economy and traffic congestion as two priorities.

However, the question as it was posed can be deceiving. That same poll also asked how much progress had been made in the respondent's community on these same five issues. Subtracting the difference between "very important" and "a lot of progress," the public collective perception highlights the frustration about traffic congestion. In regard to traffic congestion, that number is 64 percent (69 percent minus 5 percent, respectively). The other percentages ranged from 46 percent (economic growth) to 26 percent (sprawl). The public perceives traffic congestion as the most frustrating of the five problems.

A little over one year later, over 800 respondents were asked about the ability of the newly elected governor, Jim McGreevey, to successfully manage traffic congestion, cut government taxes, protect open space, cut government waste, and improve public education. The public had little confidence that the new governor could avoiding raising taxes (only 33 percent felt he could) or that he could decrease congestion and improve the state's roads (only 40 percent felt he could).

Policies and actions by several state governments, not-for-profit organizations, and some businesses aim to overcome the consequences of congestion and sprawl. New Jersey has been among the leaders of these efforts, trying to

1 End unlimited new highway construction.
2 Increase alternative travel modes (heavy rail, light rail, bicycle, and walking).
3 Design, build, and rebuild to provide people and businesses that allow people to live, work, and recreate more sustainably.
4 Target research to test which policies are more effective.

In the 1970s, Governor Brendan Byrne took action on reducing new road construction and adding transit options. In 1971, the NJTA proposed the Alfred E. Driscoll Expressway, which was to begin near exit 8A in South Brunswick in Middlesex County and run southeast to the Garden State Parkway south of exit 80 in Toms River. The environmental impact statement, a new tool at that time, supported the project with data obtained from local officials and planning boards. However, after finding widespread public and political opposition to the project in Middlesex, Monmouth, and Ocean counties, Governor Byrne halted the project. The state held the land for the project until 1979, but the governor insisted that the project would cause serious land use and environmental problems. A sad outcome of this stance was that later Governor Byrne would not be invited to Governor Driscoll's funeral.[62]

Two additional interstate projects slated for New Jersey did not see the light of day due to state and local political pressure.[63] The first was I-695, a 3.5-mile extension that would cut through the farmlands of Hopewell and Montgomery Townships, and suburban Princeton to connect I-95 to I-287. The proposal was shelved in 1980, and the federal funds were reallocated for other road projects in the same area.[64] The second project canceled was

I-895, a 6.4-mile extension planned to connect I-95 in Bucks Country, Pennsylvania, to I-295 near Burlington. Federal funding for that project was reallocated in 1981.

Building a Transit Alternative

In 2006, Governor John Corzine dedicated the NJ Transit (NJT) office complex in Newark to Louis Gambaccini. The governor described Gambaccini as "visionary, dedicated, and passionate,"[65] and we would add that Gambaccini's knowledge about mass transit was astonishing, from broad polices to station-by-station details. Governor Byrne chose Gambaccini as the New Jersey Commissioner of Transportation in 1979. Rather than walk into his new job with a solution, Commissioner Gambaccini and his staff wrote a set of white papers, one of which was aptly labeled "the horror story." It was sufficiently alarming and compelling that the state created NJ Transit, the first statewide public transit agency in the United States.

Gambaccini inherited a system of underfunded and uncoordinated freight railroad lines, limited transit services, and private bus companies that were failing economically. NJT began operating buses in 1982 and a rail system in 1983. A senior fellow at the Edward J. Bloustein School of Planning and Public Policy for many years, Gambaccini was more than willing to share his experiences. He told us that his goal was to build an interconnected heavy and light rail system and tie them to bus lines. The rail stations were key hubs for these interconnections, and the state needed to work with Amtrak to make sure that the rail lines were federally maintained. He noted the critical importance of maintaining the Port Authority Trans-Hudson (PATH) service into New York City.

NJT is the largest publicly operated transportation system and third largest provider of rail and bus service in the United States. The magnitude of its operations are impressive.[66] In 2017, NJT provided 514,000 bus passenger trips, 307,000 rail, 80,000 light rail and 5,000 on-demand passenger trips during an average week and another 700,000 total trips on an average Saturday/Sunday. It served 252 bus routes with more than 16,000 bus stops in 385 of the state's 565 municipalities. It operated three light rail lines and twelve commuter rail lines with 162 rail stations and sixty light rail stations in 116 municipalities.

NJT works with some private companies. Private bus companies provide about 20 percent of the service, with the NJT helping them with acquiring buses. In fiscal 2017, total NJT expenses were $2.3 billion, of which the system generated $1.1 billion, or 47 percent. A total of $948 million, or 41 percent came from federal and state reimbursements. Therein lies the challenge to providing current service levels and extending service: NJT has detailed plans, but the source of funds is problematic.

The state is committed to its part of the system but in the recent past has faced opposition from the U.S. government, which has been pressuring Amtrak to be financially independent and New Jersey to pay a larger share of the cost of a new tunnel between the state and New York's Pennsylvania Station. In February 2016, Weiner and Greenberg[67] polled 866 New Jersey residents about their support for repairing the over-100-year-old tunnels, adding a new tunnel under the Hudson River, and repairing two of the worst rail bridges in the United States (the Portal Bridge across the Hackensack River at Kearney and Secaucus, and the Dock Bridge across the Passaic River at Newark and Harrison). The respondents' support for public spending is summarized here.

- Building new and repairing tunnels between New York and New Jersey: 40 percent
- Improving education: 86 percent
- Improving access to health care: 77 percent
- Improving roads for auto and truck traffic: 75 percent
- Limiting property taxes: 69 percent
- Protecting open space: 61 percent

As these results show, there is far more support for improving education, access to health care, improving roads for cars and trucks, limiting property taxes, and protecting open space than for improving the rail system. On a 4-point scale, only 31 percent felt that the weakened rail tunnel system merited a "most support" response. When probed about whether they supported a user's fee to pay for tunnel repairs and additions, 54 percent favored a user's fee. However, this response disproportionately reflected people who did not ride the trains; those who wanted the repairs and new tunnels disproportionately did ride them. In short, the public as a whole has not as thoroughly accepted the need to support rail as they have other assets that are more dispersed across the state.

Although it is critical that New Jersey residents support public transit, the more immediate challenge is the federal government. History has an interesting story to tell about American politics. Although the Eisenhower administration was remarkably popular, it understood that Congress and the public would be more supportive of building an interstate highway system if defense was an explicit part of the mandate. Governor Driscoll was also careful to explicitly address the defense objective of the New Jersey Turnpike. As a result, the federal government has contributed 50 to 90 percent of interstate highway construction costs. Beginning with $25 billion from general funds, the costs were slowly shifted to a gasoline tax, which has steadily risen under federal leadership of both parties.

The gas tax is not popular, but all efforts to permanently eliminate it have failed. In 1983, a small proportion of the gas tax was dedicated to rail, and the mass transit portion has since risen to about 13 percent of the tax collection revenue.[68] Amtrak in general and New Jersey with the longest span of track in the Northeast corridor have disproportionately benefited from federal support. Amtrak's mandate requires that it serve every state. It has tried to gain wider geographical support by sponsoring new rail projects in California, Texas, and Florida, but not all the states have been receptive.[69-72] We do not believe that Amtrak can come close to achieving self-sufficiency without continuing to strongly support its Acela Express and Northeast Regional Services.

Rail service is vital, and it is much safer than transit buses and automobiles, and more reliable and cheaper per passenger mile. Research has shown that people who use rail service are more likely to meet the recommended minimum daily walking standards.[73] Studies show that riders walk to the train or bus on their journey to work, accumulating twenty to forty minutes during these trips. Of course, this changed in many places when COVID-19 struck and people worked at home. Nevertheless, some political conservatives want the federal subsidies to end and the systems to be sold. Private companies might upgrade service in some areas, but they doubtless would eliminate other services or charge more than Amtrak.[72,74].

Transportation with Health in Mind

Designing and building a healthier transportation landscape requires fresh ideas and the cooperation of local governments and not-for-profit organizations (e.g., Robert Wood Johnson Foundation, the Congress of

New Urbanism, the Active Living Network, the American Public Health Association, Smart Growth America, the Sierra Club, the Environmental Defense Fund, the Service Transportation Policy Project, and more). The premise for involving these players is that at least some of the health problems associated with the lack of physical activity among Americans is attributable to the fact that we have too few opportunities for daily exercise, especially walking and biking. Table 3.4 summarizes some of the ways that good planning and design can help improve the health of the public.

Some of these options will fail, but it is important to remain open-minded rather than skeptical. For example, food pantries and schools can by supplied by local farms; restaurants can contribute food they cannot sell. Old brownfield sites may be able to be converted to new food factories, and many people can be aided in growing their own food.[75] These are appealing options, but it is imperative that local health officials monitor food quality to be sure there is no environmental contamination (e.g., from lead chips falling from old lead-painted structures or contaminated soils around old industrial sites) or spoilage (e.g., outdated, poorly stored or refrigerated, or otherwise mishandled).[76]

Motorized scooters appear to be the latest risk and opportunity for reducing automobile use. In November 2018, author Michael Greenberg was sideswiped by a motorized scooter while walking to an American Public Health Association meeting in San Diego. The police officer who witnessed the event acknowledged that the city needed to regulate scooters because many riders had no experience in handling them so they can avoid people and automobiles, especially trucks. Smith reported that on April 23, 2019, the San Diego City Council approved rules for governing the motorized scooters and bikes that have flooded the city's streets.[77] Notably, San Diego's mayor and the city council see the scooters as a way of reducing automobile-related greenhouse gases. Smith reported that many citizens were angered by the council's decision to embrace the trend, claiming the scooters imperil public safety. Given the speed with which motorized scooters are flooding the market, it is clear that this alternative transportation option needs careful risk analysis research.[78]

Summary and Future Challenges

The United States produced about two-thirds of the world's cars during the 1950s, and America became a nation of drivers, especially after World War II

Table 3.4

Designing and Building a Healthier Landscape

Category	Options	New Jersey Context
Improve the safety of roads and bridges.	• Use traffic calming methods on roads that have a record of serious auto and pedestrian crashes. • Eliminate traffic circles. • Add overpasses and underpasses that separate motor vehicles and people. • Add signs requiring automobiles to stop and allow walkers to cross streets. • Encourage and test new modes of transportation.	New Jersey has among the highest or the highest proportion of pedestrian and auto fatalities.
Take advantage of rail and bus access opportunities by building transit-oriented developments with dense concentrations of homes, stores, and services.	• Design and implement high-density settlements near rail, light rail, and bus stops. • Consider redeveloping brownfields and grayfields into multiuse commercial and residential developments, art galleries/museums, and recreation facilities. • Accommodate ethnic diversity. • Establish economical ferry services. • Experiment with personal transportation options, evaluating for risk and opportunities.	Rahway, Elizabeth, New Brunswick, and Metropark are examples of transit-oriented developments. Use brownfield and grayfield sites when possible.
Build physical, social, and cultural connections between cites, suburbs, and rural areas.	• Preserve open space. • Preserve watershed areas, especially near wells and potable surface water sites. • Build relationships between local, suburban, and rural food sources and markets, especially schools, health care, and community groups. • Plant water- and fire-resistant vegetation, especially in vulnerable locations.	New Jersey was an early adopter of many of these options, including urban gardens, gleaning programs, and urban farm markets on selected days.

SOURCES: Frumkin et al. (2004)[42]; Newman and Kenworthy (1999)[49]; McCann and DeLille (2000)[52]; Dannenberg et al. (2011)[53]; Frank (2000)[60]; Vallianatos et al. (2004)[75]; Greenberg and Schneider (2017)[76]; Smith (2019)[77]; Greenfield (2019).[78]

when federal highway funds stimulated the growth of suburban development. This chapter demonstrates that postwar policies stimulated middle-class wealth, allowing many to access homeownership for the first time. Funding for new roads opened up new tracts of land for employers to move to larger spaces, and land became available for large prefabricated developments, massive shopping malls, and other amenities that people wanted. Federal, state, and local policies all pointed Americans toward the suburbs and away from cities. As a result, the suburbs and the Sunbelt expanded, and many Northeast and Midwest cities shrank, leaving many underprivileged and underserved individuals behind.

Health statistics show that Americans walk less and weigh more than they did seventy years ago. It is undeniable that at least some of this is the result of the public policies that underfunded public transit and supported roadbuilding and suburbanization. Using data between 1999 and 2009, Buehler and Pucher found that only about 10 percent of U.S. daily trips were by walking or biking compared with 51 percent in the Netherlands, 34 percent in Denmark, and 34 percent in Germany.[79] Canada and Australia, both large countries like the United States, now resemble the United States in automobile dominance with only 12 and 6 percent of trips, respectively, without a motorized vehicle. It is a simple fact that many Americans simply cannot get from one place to another easily without encountering transportation limitations. Those who walk or bike may encounter roadways that endanger both motorists and pedestrians.

Not-for-profit organizations, some elected officials, and individuals have taken on the challenge of slowing down and reversing these trends, which have now been in existence for more than seven decades. They face the following challenges.

- During a recession or what elected officials think might become a recession, government and private individuals are prone to stimulate the construction industry to create jobs. State transportation departments have a list of road projects on their shelves waiting for the opportunity to build. Those interested in increasing nonautomotive transportation options need to be sure that projects that will stimulate safe nonauto options are also sitting on shelves waiting to be suggested and acted on.
- The federal government continues to threaten Amtrak's funding. If Amtrak is unable to continue strong service in New Jersey and

along the Northeast corridor line, NJT will not be able to continue its current level of service. This means the state economy, as well as other state assets that directly and indirectly affect health, will be in peril.

- Influential political insiders have a propensity to offer simple solutions to complex problems. Relatively simple ideas like planting more trees and preserving green space, and adding safer sidewalks, off-street parking, and safer street crossings are usually politically acceptable. However, these need to be supplemented with struc-tural solutions such as mixed-use zoning, transit-oriented develop-ments, light and heavier transit, traffic-calming techniques, and other more expensive projects that some people will oppose. Civic organizations and academic experts need to be available to testify before decision-makers about the true complexity behind New Jersey's commitment to transit and nonauto options.
- The transportation research community must help to counter the belief that political ideology rather than scientifically conducted studies should be the key to achieving a better understanding of travel options. It needs to be able to reach out to key players in New Jersey's health community and work together with them regarding the sprawl-related issues discussed in this chapter.
- Environmental justice in the collective mind of many people is associated with hazardous waste sites, air pollution, water pollu-tion, and other risks identified in the 1970s and 1980s. However, many of the worst environmental justice consequences have resulted from the spread of people and jobs across the landscape, leaving pockets of poverty and contamination that are invisible to many of us. A major challenge will be to monitor the environmen-tal and social justice issues, including many that result from the allocation of money for transportation.

The years 1946 to 1964 presented a unique era when the U.S. economy flourished and many Americans perceived that even the sky was not the limit. Postwar opportunities allowed many to flourish and establish a high quality of life. The opportunities presented, however, did not come with-out consequences. Perhaps the single most difficult challenge for managing today's structural consequences is how to energize many disengaged Amer-icans into thinking less about individualism and more about the public good, including their own community's health. Only with popular commitment will New Jersey will be able to build and grow a culture of health that can significantly influence state, local, and federal agencies to consider Health in All Policies.

References

1 Breckman A. *Moving* [film], dir. Metter A. Burbank, CA: Warner Bros; 1988.
2 The postwar economy: 1945–1960. In: American history: from Revolution to Reconstruction and beyond. University of Groningen—Humanities Computing, 1994–2012. http://www.let.rug.nl/usa/outlines/history-1994/postwar-america/the-postwar-economy-1945-1960.php
3 Patton M. U.S. role in global economy declines nearly 50%. *Forbes*, February 29, 2016. https://www.forbes.com/sites/mikepatton/2016/02/29/u-s-role-in-global-economy-declines-nearly-50/
4 Voth H-J, Voigtländer N. Nazi pork and popularity: how Hitler's roads won German hearts and minds. VoxEU CEPR Policy Portal, May 22, 2014. https://cepr.org/voxeu/columns/nazi-pork-and-popularity-how-hitlers-roads-won-german-hearts-and-minds
5 PeriscopeFilm. New Jersey Turnpike Super Highway 1950s Newsreel 74752 [video]. *YouTube*, July 20, 2015, 22:32. https://www.youtube.com/watch?v=hSRhEJc3GHw
6 Driscoll A. Fourth Annual Message, Alfred E. Driscoll, Governor of New Jersey, to the Legislature, January 9, 1951. https://dspace.njstatelib.org/xmlui/bitstream/handle/10929/16762/1951.pdf
7 Blackwell J. 1949: Highway of dreams. *Capital Century,* January 18, 2008. http://www.capitalcentury.com/1949.html
8 Reif C. Taconic Parkway among "most dangerous, deadly places in NY," website says. *Yorktown Daily Voice,* January 15, 2017. https://dailyvoice.com/new-york/yorktown/lifestyle/taconic-parkway-among-most-dangerous-deadly-places-in-ny-website-says/696370/
9 Monroe L. The deadliest road in New York is one you'll want to avoid. *Only in Your State,* January 8, 2022. https://www.onlyinyourstate.com/new-york/deadliest-road-ny/
10 Manuscript Group 1544, New Jersey Turnpike Collection. In: Guide to the New Jersey Turnpike Collection 1950–2003, MG 1544. New Jersey Historical Society. https://jerseyhistory.org/guide-to-the-new-jersey-turnpike-collection1950-2003/
11 Gillespie AK, Rockland MA. *Looking for America on the New Jersey Turnpike.* New Brunswick, NJ: Rutgers University Press; 1989.
12 New Jersey Turnpike Authority. Travel tools: service areas & commuter lots. Updated 2022. https://www.njta.com/travel-resources/service-areas-commuter-lots
13 NJ Turnpike Interchange 6 to 9 widening program. Program Documents. New Jersey Turnpike Authority. http://www.njturnpikewidening.com/index.php
14 Shipkowski B. Turnpike widening from exit 6 to 9 nearly complete. *Associated Press/My Central Jersey,* October 23, 2014. https://www.mycentraljersey.com/story/news/local/middlesex-county/2014/10/23/nj-turnpike-new-brunswick/17775233/

15 Colimore E. What a relief extra lanes on the N.J. Turnpike are. *Philadelphia Inquirer*, November 25, 2014. https://www.inquirer.com/philly/news/new_jersey /20141126_Snow_and_rain_may_stymie_traffic__but_not_any_NJ_turnpike _bottleneck.html

16 Higgs L. Traffic, toll revenues set record pace on Parkway, Turnpike. *NJ.com*, March 3, 2017. https://www.nj.com/traffic/2017/03/parkway_turnpike_break _predictions_for_traffic_and.html

17 Davis M. A tax by any other name: NJ pays one-fifth of all tolls in U.S. *App/USA Today*, October 23, 2015. https://www.app.com/story/news/traffic/commuting /2015/10/23/nj-tolls-highest/73819930/

18 Martucci B. 14 U.S. cities with the worst traffic & longest commute times. *Money Crashers*, August 9, 2022. https://www.moneycrashers.com/worst-us-cities-traffic -commute-time/

19 Higgs L. These are the 25 worst traffic hotspots in America. Four are here. *NJ.com*, October 9, 2017. https://www.nj.com/traffic/2017/10/these_are_the_25_worst _traffic_hotspots_in_america_four_are_here.html

20 Salant JD. Here's a big reason truckers may hate New Jersey. *NJ.com*, October 22, 2018. https://www.nj.com/politics/2018/10/how_much_extra_truckers_pay _each_year_to_sit_in_je.html

21 Quinn P, Breeze J. Planning the final-mile: the New Jersey Turnpike corridor. Colliers International, October 18, 2018. https://www.colliers.com/en/research /2018-us-industrial-planning-the-final-mile-nj-corridor

22 Fishman R. The American metropolis at century's end: past and future influences. *Housing Policy Debate*. 2000;11(1):199–213. doi:10.1080/10511482.2000.9521367

23 Straight line diagrams. 2009 ed. Trenton, NJ: New Jersey Department of Transportation. https://www.state.nj.us/transportation/refdata/sldiag/

24 Glass M. These are the 10 most dangerous roads in the US. MoneyWise, December 19, 2021. https://www.yahoo.com/video/10-most-dangerous-roads-us-160000716 .html#:~:text=The%20combination%20of%20high%20speed,a%20total%20 of%20209%20deaths.

25 New Jersey Map Collection. *Geology.com*. https://geology.com/state-map/new -jersey.shtml

26 Schwartz H. Fuel implications of suburb-to-suburb commuting. *The Fuse*, January 29, 2018. http://energyfuse.org/fuel-implications-of-suburb-to-suburb -commuting/

27 U.S. Census Bureau. Historical census of housing tables: homeownership. 2020. Updated October 8, 2021. https://www.census.gov/data/tables/time-series/dec /coh-owner.html

28 Rosenberg M. History and overview of Levittown Housing Developments. *ThoughtCo*, July 3, 2019. https://www.thoughtco.com/levittown-long-island-1435787

29 Torres J, Singer A. Levittown, PA and the "Northern Promised Land that wasn't." *History News Network*, February 24, 2019. https://historynewsnetwork.org/article /171333

30 Helphand KI. McUrbia: the 1950s and the birth of the contemporary American landscape. *Places*. 1988;5(2):40–49. http://escholarship.org/uc/item/84s22575

31 Ura A. Dallas-Fort Worth Metro area saw biggest population growth in Texas in 2018. *Texas Tribune*, April 18, 2019. https://www.texastribune.org/2019/04/18 /dallas-fort-worth-metro-area-saw-biggest-2018-texas-population-growth/

32 Berry BJL. *Commercial Structure and Commercial Blight: Retail Patterns and Processes in the City of Chicago*. Chicago: Department of Geography, University of Chicago; 1963.

33 Petro G. Shopping malls aren't dying—they're evolving. *Forbes*, April 5, 2019. https://www.forbes.com/sites/gregpetro/2019/04/05/shopping-malls-arent-dying -theyre-evolving/

34 Greenberg MR. *Siting Noxious Facilities: Integrating Location Economics and Risk Analysis to Protect Environmental Health and Investments*. New York: Routledge; 2018.

35 Staples JH. Urban renewal: a comparative study of twenty-two cities, 1950–1960. *West Polit Q*. 1970;23(2):294–304. doi:10.1177/106591297002300205

36 Mieszkowski P, Mills ES. The causes of metropolitan suburbanization. *J Econ Perspect*. 1993;7(3):135–147. doi:10.1257/jep.7.3.135

37 Kopecky KA, Suen RMH. A quantitative analysis of suburbanization and the diffusion of the automobile. *Int Econ Rev*. 2010;51(4):1003–1037. doi:10.1111/ j.1468-2354.2010.00609.x

38 Baum-Snow N. Did highways cause suburbanization? *Q J Econ*. 2007;122(2): 775–805. doi:10.1162/qjec.122.2.775

39 Boustan LP. Was postwar suburbanization "white flight"? Evidence from the Black Migration. *Q J Econ*. 2010;125(1):417–443. doi:10.1162/qjec.2010.125.1.417

40 Frey WH. Central city white flight: racial and nonracial causes. *Am Sociol Rev*. 1979;44(3):425–448. doi:10.2307/2094885

41 Ravitch D. Social science and social policy: the "white flight" controversy. *Public Interest*. 1978;51:125–149.

42 Frumkin H, Frank LD, Jackson R. *Urban Sprawl and Public Health: Designing, Planning, and Building for Healthy Communities*. Washington, DC: Island Press; 2004.

43 Cockerham WC. *Social Causes of Health and Disease*. Malden, MA: Polity Press; 2007.

44 Berrigan D, Troiano RP. The association between urban form and physical activity in U.S. adults. *Am J Prev Med*. 2002;23(2 Suppl):74–79. doi:10.1016/ s0749-3797(02)00476-2

45 Semenza JC, Rubin CH, Falter KH, et al. Heat-related deaths during the July 1995 heat wave in Chicago. *N Engl J Med*. 1996;335(2):84–90. doi:10.1056/NEJM19960 7113350203

46 Rathbone DB. *Controlling Road Rage: A Literature Review and Pilot Study*. Washington, DC: InterTrans Group; 1999. https://rosap.ntl.bts.gov/view/dot/14155

47 Kaplan GA, Pamuk ER, Lynch JW, Cohen RD, Balfour JL. Inequality in income and mortality in the United States: analysis of mortality and potential pathways. *BMJ*. 1996;312(7037):999–1003. doi:10.1136/bmj.312.7037.999

48 Wilson WJ. *The Truly Disadvantaged: The Inner City, the Underclass, and Public Policy*. Chicago: University of Chicago Press; 2012.

49 Newman P, Kenworthy JR. *Sustainability and Cities: Overcoming Automobile Dependence*. Washington, DC: Island Press; 1999.

50 Wing JS. Asthma in the inner city—a growing public health concern in the United States. *J Asthma*. 1993;30(6):427–430. doi:10.3109/02770909309056750

51 Whitman S, Good G, Donoghue ER, et al. Mortality in Chicago attributed to the July 1995 heat wave. *Am J Public Health*. 1997;87(9):1515–1518. doi:10.2105/ AJPH.87.9.1515

52 McCann B, DeLille B. *Mean Streets 2000: Pedestrian Safety, Health and Federal Transportation.* Washington, DC: Surface Transportation Policy Project; 2000. http://www.transact.org/PDFs/ms2000/ms2000.pdf

53 Dannenberg A, Frumkin H, Jackson R, eds. *Making Healthy Places: Designing and Building for Health, Well-Being, and Sustainability.* Washington, DC: Island Press; 2011.

54 Duany A, Plater-Zyberk E, Speck J. *Suburban Nation: The Rise of Sprawl and the Decline of the American Dream.* New York: North Point Press; 2000.

55 National Research Council. *Air Pollution, the Automobile, and Public Health.* Washington, DC: National Academies Press; 1988. doi:10.17226/1033

56 Pope CA, Thun MJ, Namboodiri MM, et al. Particulate air pollution as a predictor of mortality in a prospective study of U.S. adults. *Am J Respir Crit Care Med.* 1995;151(3):669–674. doi:10.1164/ajrccm/151.3_Pt_1.669

57 Centers for Disease Control and Prevention. Motor-vehicle safety: a 20th century public health achievement. *MMWR Morb Mortal Wkly Rep.* 1999;48(18):369–374. https://www.cdc.gov/mmwr/preview/mmwrhtml/mm4818a1.htm

58 Thompson PD, Buchner D, Pina IL, et al. Exercise and physical activity in the prevention and treatment of atherosclerotic cardiovascular disease: a statement from the Council on Clinical Cardiology (Subcommittee on Exercise, Rehabilitation, and Prevention) and the Council on Nutrition, Physical Activity, and Metabolism (Subcommittee on Physical Activity). Circulation. 2003 Jun 24; 107(24):3109–16. doi: 10.1161/01.CIR.0000075572.40158.77. PMID: 12821592.

59 Centers for Disease Control and Prevention. Surgeon General's report on physical activity and health. *JAMA.* 1996;276(7):522. doi:10.1001/jama.1996.03540070018010

60 Frank LD. Land use and transportation interaction: implications on public health and quality of life. *J Plan Educ Res.* 2000;20(1):6–22. doi:10.1177/0739456001 28992564

61 Caro RA. *The Power Broker: Robert Moses and the Fall of New York.* New York: Alfred A. Knopf; 1974.

62 Kim S, Zafari Z, Bellanger M, Muennig PA. Cost-effectiveness of capping freeways for use as parks: the New York Cross-Bronx Expressway case study. *Am J Public Health.* 2018;108(3):379–384. doi:10.2105/AJPH.2017.304243

63 Center for Public Interest Polling/Eagleton Poll, Poll #130, January 2001. Eagleton Poll Archive, Rutgers University. https://eagleton.libraries.rutgers.edu /pollDetail.php?PollNum=130

64 Nordheimer J. Traffic jams around Princeton rekindle a highway debate. *New York Times,* February 12, 1995. https://www.nytimes.com/1995/02/12/nyregion /traffic-jams-around-princeton-rekindle-a-highway-debate.html

65 Stessel D. NJ Transit Headquarters dedicated to honor transportation visionary Louis J. Gambaccini [press release]. NJ Transit, September 13, 2006. https://www .njtransit.com/press-releases/nj-transit-hq-dedicated-honor-transportation -visionary-louis-j-gambaccini

66 Department of Compliance. NJ TRANSIT Facts at a Glance FY 2017; 2018.

67 Weiner MD, Greenberg MR. The Hudson Tunnel Project: exploring public opinion support for public funding mechanisms for critical infrastructure. *Case Stud Transp Policy.* 2018;6(2):265–278. doi:10.1016/J.CSTP.2018.04.005

68 Davis J. Why is the mass transit account less solvent than the highway account? ENO Center for Transportation, April 11, 2019. https://www.enotrans.org/article /why-is-the-mass-transit-account-less-solvent-than-the-highway-account/

69 Amtrak. *FY 2018 Company Profile*. Washington, DC; 2019.

70 Nice DC. *Amtrak: The History and Politics of a National Railroad*. Boulder, CO: Lynne Rienner; 1998.

71 Wilner FN. *Amtrak: Past, Present, Future*. Omaha, NE: Simmons-Boardman; 2012.

72 Baron DP. Distributive politics and the persistence of Amtrak. *J Politics*. 1990; 52(3):883–913. doi:10.2307/2131831

73 Greenberg M, Renne J, Lane R, Zupan J. Physical activity and use of suburban train stations: an exploratory analysis. *J Public Transp*. 2005;8(3):89–116. doi:10.5038/2375-0901.8.3.5

74 Curley R. Trump proposes big cuts to Amtrak and other rail projects. *Business Traveller*, April 4, 2019. https://www.businesstraveller.com/business-travel/2019 /04/04/trump-proposes-big-cuts-to-amtrak-and-other-rail-projects/

75 Vallianatos M, Gottlieb R, Haase MA. Farm-to-school: strategies for, urban health, combatting sprawl, and establishing a community food systems approach. *J Plan Educ Res*. 2004;23(4):414–423. doi:10.1177/0739456X04264765

76 Greenberg MR, Schneider D. *Urban Planning and Public Health: A Critical Partnership*. Washington, DC: American Public Health Association; 2017.

77 Smith JE. San Diego approves rules for electric scooters as angry residents crowd City Hall. *San Diego Union-Tribune*, April 23, 2019. https://www.sandiego uniontribune.com/news/politics/story/2019-04-23/san-diego-approvals-rules-for -dockless-scooters-as-angry-residents-crowd-city-hall

78 Greenfield J. Not-so-easy riders. *Chicago Reader*, August 14, 2019. https://chicago reader.com/columns-opinion/not-so-easy-riders/

79 Buehler R, Pucher J. Walking and cycling in Western Europe and the United States: trends, policies, and lessons. *TR News*. 2012;280(May–June):34–42. https://onlinepubs.trb.org/onlinepubs/trnews/trnews280WesternEurope.pdf

4

Fixing Environmental Inequities

Cancer Alley

Whether it is New Jersey, Louisiana, Texas, or another state, the label "Cancer Alley" is an unfriendly one—the proverbial tarring and feathering of a location. Who would want to move to a place with high cancer rates? Who would invest their resources to establish a business there? This chapter has four objectives:

1 Summarize the origin of the Cancer Alley label.
2 Examine why occupational and environmental exposures were assumed to be the primary cause of cancer deaths.
3 Offer alternative explanations, such as personal behaviors, migration, and delays in identifying and treating the disease.
4 Review the response of state an officials and the public's concern about environmental protection.

Cancer Alley

We do not know who coined the label Cancer Alley. During the 1970s, several people pointed the finger at Michael Greenberg, the first author, and he pointed it back at reporters—at least one from New Jersey and one from Washington, DC. These reporters had heard, read, and even written about New Jersey as Cancer Alley, but none would not take responsibility for the epithet. We still hear the state identified with the term. However, a web search today will identify the area between Baton Rouge and New Orleans—a stretch of Louisiana along the Mississippi River with a dense concentration of chemical plants and refineries—as the current Cancer Alley; Brendan Byrne, who was governor of New Jersey during that Cancer Alley era, later laughed when told that another unlucky state now owned the stigmatizing label.

During the 1970s and early 1980s, several individuals and company representatives contacted Michael Greenberg with concerns about the widely publicized Cancer Alley label attached to New Jersey. Some wanted to know if they should avoid moving to the state; others wanted to know if they should move out. Not only was Cancer Alley a nasty slur, it was inaccurate, as Greenberg demonstrated in the article "Does New Jersey Cause Cancer?"[1] As he explained, the death rates failed to recognize the long latency period associated with the majority of cancers. Indeed, by the time the notion of Cancer Alley became public, the reality of higher cancer death rates in New Jersey no longer existed. Yet as late as the 1990s, Dona Schneider, the second author, was still receiving calls from concerned parents about whether their child was at risk of "catching" cancer because it had been diagnosed in another child in their community (usually in the form of brain cancer or leukemia). It was clear that adverse publicity had stoked fear among New Jersey residents, and it had more impact than academic papers, health education, or public health messages about the label's inaccuracy.

The evidence that led to the original Cancer Alley designation was a result of the computer revolution. At the National Institutes of Health (NIH), scientists gained access to large mainframe computers that could rapidly count, calculate, and map information at local geographical scales for the first time. In 1975, the National Cancer Institute published a 729-page data book that listed the cancer death rates in the United States by county for the aggregated period of 1950 through 1969.[2] Michael Greenberg received a copy of the data book from a member of the NCI research

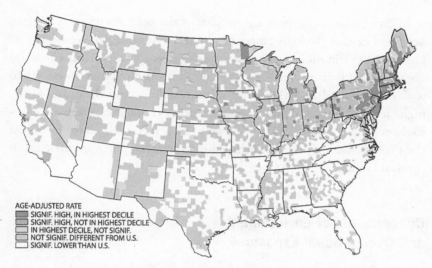

AGE-ADJUSTED RATE
■ SIGNIF. HIGH, IN HIGHEST DECILE
■ SIGNIF. HIGH, NOT IN HIGHEST DECILE
□ IN HIGHEST DECILE, NOT SIGNIF.
□ NOT SIGNIF. DIFFERENT FROM U.S.
□ SIGNIF. LOWER THAN U.S.

FIGURE 4.1 Total white female cancer mortality by county, 1950–1969. (*Source:* Mason et al. (1975).[3])

team: the size of the book was imposing, with endless tables of white male and female deaths, and the age-adjusted death rates for the various cancers that occurred in each of the counties in the United States. The county-level data were geocoded so that New Jersey was state 34. Each county had a three-digit tag that followed the state geocode, so Atlantic County appeared as 34001, Bergen County as 34003, and so on. With an average of 850 numbers on each page of the tome, the data book was too massive for the information in it to be available to the vast majority of potential readers.

The results published in the data book did not become the grist for the Cancer Alley label until the NCI published an atlas of cancer mortality.[2] The maps in the atlas were provocative, with red and orange signifying high cancer death rates. The colors identified New Jersey as part, maybe the core, of a ribbon of cancer deaths stretching from New England through Pennsylvania along Route 95 (see also chapter 3). Figure 4.1 illustrates the Cancer Alley pattern for total cancer deaths among white females.

The text in the atlas was also provocative. For example, the results and discussion begin as follows: "A cluster of high rates in the Northeast (New Jersey, Southern New York, Connecticut, Rhode Island, and Massachusetts)" (ix).[3] The text also pointed out places with high death rates for particular cancers, including New Jersey for cancers of the large intestine and rectum, larynx, female breast, and male bladder.

Michael Greenberg spent a good part of the next seven years trying to demonstrate that the high cancer death rates that tarnished New Jersey as Cancer Alley did not exist by the time the atlas appeared. This effort did not sit well with many New Jersey residents who asserted that he was in bed with industry. Policy-makers sought information about the causes of the high rates and became concerned about identifying those causes and effectively managing cancer-related illnesses in New Jersey and elsewhere across the United States. These concerns led to examining potential toxic exposures and more.

Concerns about Environmental and Occupational Exposures

Anyone looking at the cancer atlas maps and recognizing the industrial history of New Jersey (see chapter 2) could easily assume that industrial contamination was the cause of at least some of the high cancer death rates. Indeed, many could still see, hear, and smell the dark side of the state's industrialization legacy. The strongest link between the state's industrial legacy and its higher cancer mortality rates might be from Salem County, where the death rates for male (but not female) bladder cancer were more than elevated. In NCI analyses,[2–3] Salem County had the highest male bladder cancer rate in the United States, and seventeen of the twenty other New Jersey counties were among the highest decile of male bladder cancer rates. Those results were widely touted as evidence of the role of carcinogenic chemicals causing environmental cancers. The elevated male bladder cancer death rates were later shown to be related to chemical dyes in the male-only workplace.[4]

Concerns about pollution causing cancer focused on chemical agents, but also the overall contamination of our air, water, and land. Air quality has been a challenge in New Jersey for well over a century. In 2020 New Jersey had over 9 million residents, yet no city in state had anywhere close to one-half million people. Rather, the state has a dense, overall distribution of people, industry, and mobile sources of air pollution that are never far away from our homes. Some of the most affluent New Jersey suburbs include portions of the heavily traveled New Jersey Turnpike, Route 80, and other interstate highways (see chapter 3). Because of these concerns, New Jersey, along with neighboring New York City and Philadelphia, made efforts at reducing air emissions as early as the 1950s.[5,6] In 1954, New Jersey adopted one of the first statewide air pollution laws, the Air Pollution Control Act,[7] which mandated control strategies for open burning in 1956, and later for coal combustion and incineration.[8,9]

Stern[10,11] summarized the total suspended particulates (TSP) measurements in ambient air across the nation from 1953 to 1957 using data from the U.S. National Air Sampling Network. TSP was high in multiple places, including many parts of New Jersey. In fact, state officials and urban residents across the state at that time must have personally experienced significant soot and haze (along with breathing problems for those who were more sensitive), leading them to have concerns about air pollution. Many would have reasonably assumed that urban air pollution caused cancer. In response, the New Jersey Legislature strengthened its air pollution law in 1967, before the United States passed the Clean Air Act of 1970. The law set ambient air quality and new source performance standards, and controlled sulfur content in fuels.[12]

Another explanation for the high cancer rates linked to pollution was leaking landfills and industrial waste management sites. In New Jersey, as in many other places, urbanization required residential waste management from either government or private haulers. Industry often had its own disposal sites or contracts with private haulers. Initially, heavy deposits of waste filled the Hackensack Meadowlands in the northern part of the state and in the Pinelands in southern New Jersey. Lawsuits at the federal level used the Commerce Clause (Article 1, Section 8, Clause 3 of the U.S. Constitution) to block efforts by New Jersey to prevent outside haulers from depositing waste in the state.

Not until the creation of the New Jersey Department of Environmental Protection in 1970 did the state as a whole have much power to control waste management. Perhaps the most egregious case of land contamination was the Kin-Buc Landfill, located in Edison, New Jersey, less than six miles from our own offices. Opened in the late 1940s, it received 70 million gallons of liquid toxic waste. It also received industrial solid hazardous and non-hazardous waste, which it mixed with household garbage. On several occasions, the landfill caught on fire. In one instance, an explosion killed a bulldozer operator who had been compacting hazardous waste. The 220-acre site was planning to increase in size until state and federal officials intervened in 1976, closing the eyesore and beginning to remediate it. The closure was completed in 2002, and the U.S. Environmental Protection Agency (EPA) continues activities there for operation and maintenance.[13]

When the Cancer Alley idea first became prominent, people living near landfills or throughways where garbage trucks passed would have been justified if they believed that the waste materials were dangerous to their health. The odors alone were horrendous. Public pressure to deal with pollution led the New Jersey state legislature to pass the Public Health Priority Funding Act of 1977, stating,

> The Legislature finds and declares that there exists in New Jersey a serious and increasing incidence of various communicable and chronic diseases such as cancer, hypertension, heart disease, diabetes, venereal disease, alcoholism and drug abuse which requires a continuing commitment of public health personnel and resources; and that there has been in recent years a diminished financial support for agencies engaged in providing primary prevention programs.[14]

The law required adopting a sanitary code, but implementation remained primarily in the hands of selected local governments and private industry. When Michael Greenberg served on a state panel examining solutions for closing landfills during the mid-1980s, he learned that there were well over 1,000 landfills across the state, some within five miles of his house, that he knew nothing about. Given the context of the time, a resident of New Jersey would have to have been deaf, dumb, and blind not to conclude that exposure to occupational toxins and pollution of our air, water, and land were major contributors to the state's high cancer rates.

Alternative Explanations for Cancer Mortality

Other explanations for New Jersey's high cancer death rates were suggested, some of which were more difficult to accept than others. For example, some hypothesized that viruses were responsible for many environmental cancers. This hypothesis was taken seriously by many researchers and the public; when President Richard Nixon declared war on cancer in the National Cancer Act of 1971, considerable resources were provided to investigate this possibility. Another hypothesis was that New Jersey's hot and humid summers caused the production of aflatoxins that contaminated foods and caused cancer. Michael Greenberg recalls participating in a radio show during which one of the participants insisted that New Jersey's humidity was a major cause, despite many other states having equally high humidity and the cancers he pointed to as evidence being on the decline.

The strongest evidence against the idea that occupational toxins and environmental pollution were the major causes of cancer came from two distinguished British cancer researchers, Sir Richard Doll and Richard Peto.[15] The Office of Technology Assessment of the U.S. Congress funded them to prepare a review of the major causes of cancer. Their credibility was further enhanced by the reality that they also worked on the relationship between radiation and leukemia,[16] asbestos and lung cancer,[17] and alcohol and breast cancer,[18] even though they were best known for studying the relationship between cigarette smoking and lung cancer.[18] In other words, Doll and Peto had immense credibility. These two senior epidemiologists' best estimates were that 6 percent of cancers could be attributed to occupation and pollution (range: <3 percent to 13 percent). By contrast, they attributed 35 percent of cancers to diet and 30 percent to smoking tobacco.[15]

Detailed smoking histories are common today, but such information was not readily available before 1970. Instead, researchers used epidemiological studies of migrants and their first-generation children to infer differences in smoking and dietary habits. Writing for the International Agency for Research on Cancer, Kmet[19] noted how few migrant studies have been done. In regard to the significantly higher rates of cancer mortality found in New Jersey compared with elsewhere, only cancer of the esophagus showed clearly consistent findings for the migrant contribution. For cancers of the lung, large intestine and rectum, male bladder, and female breast, migrant studies showed some excess in mortality for native Europeans who moved to the United States, but for other cancers they had lower rates. In contrast to Kmet's findings, Gordon et al.[20] found no migrant effect but did point to higher cancer death rates in the Northeast and Midwest parts of the United States. Overall, the migrant hypothesis did not turn out to be a major explanation for the causes of cancer reflected in the cancer atlas.

It is important to remember that the cancer atlas focused on "white" Americans.[3] It did not consider the nonwhite population because of the wide variation of subpopulations included within that designation (see chapter 2). Yet migrant studies can be valuable epidemiological tools to gain insights about differences among populations. At least two migrant studies examined the geographical variations in cancer mortality among African Americans. The first study found marked differences between Black individuals born in the South and those born in the Northeast, Midwest, and Western parts of the United States. Even after migrating to regions with lower cancer mortality rates, Black migrants from the South carried with them the cancer mortality risks of Southern-born African Americans.[21] A second study explored diets within the group that identified as African American. It showed that the diet of the Black population born in the United States was markedly different from those who were born and migrated to the United States from the Caribbean.[22] The authors hypothesized that the lower cancer mortality rates among immigrants from the Caribbean were perhaps due to cultural, dietary, and other personal behaviors carried with them from their place of birth. Perhaps some of these behaviors, or the lack of them, protected them from developing cancers relative to native-born Black Americans.

By the time the cancer atlas appeared, the difference in cancer death rates between New Jersey and the United States was negligible, as demonstrated by a cooperative data project between Greenberg and the NCI.[23] Restructuring the age-adjusted cancer mortality data into five-year time periods, the study demonstrated that during the first time period, from 1950 to 1954, the New Jersey white male rate was 23 percent higher than the national one. By 1970 to 1974, the difference was only 10 percent higher, and the gap between the two rates was continuing to fall. For white males 35 to 54 years of age, the New Jersey rate was 20 percent higher than national rate, but the difference fell to less than 1 percent by 1970 to 1974. These results are consistent with the assertion that the nation is moving toward a more homogeneous pattern of health outcomes at the macroscale, even though there are ongoing and even growing differences at the neighborhood level because of health inequities.

Another untested hypothesis offered for the patterns in the cancer atlas was that differences in health care could account for some of the excess deaths. At the time of the Cancer Alley debate, there was no ability to answer this question. Today, large databases allow researchers with clearance to compare disease recognition and treatment across a variety of demographic indicators. Specifically, better access to diagnosis and treatment might increase the reported number of newly diagnosed cancers (cancer incidence), but it need not necessarily reflect higher cancer mortality rates. Indeed, some people are cured of their disease, and others live their lives with their disease in remission.

Recent comparisons of cancer incidence and cancer death rates further demonstrate how access to care and diagnosis might be an explanation for increasing cancer survivorship. From 2000 to 2020, the U.S. cancer death rate decreased from 196.5 to 144.1 deaths per 100,000 population.[24] The New Jersey cancer death rate in 2020 was 133.4 per 100,000 population—in other words, well below the national average.[24] Yet in terms of cancer incidence, New Jersey rates were high. The National Cancer Institute (NCI) reported that from 2014 to 2018, New Jersey ranked second among the states in cancer incidence rates, behind only Kentucky.[25] Its neighbors, New York, Pennsylvania, and Delaware, ranked 5, 7, and 8, respectively.

While the incidence of cancer continues to be high across the nation, more people than ever are surviving their cancer diagnosis. NCI reports that as of January 2019, there were an estimated 16.9 million cancer survivors in the United States.[26] In New Jersey, the prospects for surviving cancer are exceptionally good because of the state's early identification of new cases, and a health care system with the capacity to alter what once was a fatal diagnosis. In short, it is plausible that New Jersey residents, especially those with health insurance and access to good health care, understand that speed is of the essence when it comes to preventing cancer from being a killer. This implies that more New Jersey residents than those residing in neighboring states have overcome the fear of cancer and the tendency to pretend that no news is good news.[27]

Actions and Advocacy for Protecting the Public's Health

We would be hard-pressed to think of health-related issue in which residents of New Jersey have been more active than in environmental health. The Cancer Alley concern, we believe, helped stimulate this interest. It led to the establishment of a Health in All Policies (HiAP) perspective and a culture of health that understands the importance of the issues and the connections between human health and environmental protection.

As noted in chapter 2, Hall and Kerr[28] created a state green index with 256 indicators. New Jersey ranked 14 among the fifty states overall, but its overall rank was 28 in green conditions and 3 in green policy. This striking difference, unmatched across the United States, allows us to infer that the state recognizes its significant environmental issues and has made major policy efforts to deal with them. Space does not permit a full presentation of all the policy efforts designed to improve the environment in New Jersey. Instead, we focus on those aimed at reducing air pollution, improving hazardous waste management and water quality, and the creation of the New Jersey Commission on Cancer Research.

Air Pollution

New Jersey created the Department of Environmental Protection on April 22, 1970, the date coinciding with the first Earth Day. Lioy and Georgopoulos[29] estimated that between 1970 and 1975, the state created more than 200 environmental laws, regulations, and practices. Many of these were for air pollution, including

- Ambient air quality standards.
- Chemical storage facilities emission limits.
- Control of gas and particle emissions.
- Facility permits.
- Landfill emission standards.
- Motor vehicle emission requirements, including trucks.
- Smoke control.
- Stricter control of toxic air emissions.

The large number of environmental laws and policies promulgated in New Jersey was not simply a reaction to the public's environmental concerns. The state had data that demonstrated that federal regulations on air pollution were not sufficiently strong to protect human health. New Jersey began collecting air pollution data before the passage of the federal Clean Air Act of 1970. The data showed that as the industrial footprint in the state began to decline, there was a similar reduction in industrial point source emissions. Additionally, when federal legislation removing lead from gasoline passed, a reduction in atmospheric lead quickly followed. The New Jersey data were some of the most convincing provided to federal officials in support of setting the 1978 lead standard for ambient air.[30] Soot, sulfur oxides, and particulates in ambient air also declined as coal-burning technologies in homes and power plants were replaced with oil and natural gas.

New Jersey was far from a clean air state during the 1950s and 1960s. Stern[10,31] and Lioy and Georgopoulos[29] remind us that during that time we used the Ringelmann Chart of "blackness" to identify emissions sources. The coefficient of haze (COH) tool also helped identify industrial point source air emissions.[32] Our students could use their olfactory senses, the

Ringelmann Chart, and the COH tool by traversing the New Jersey Turnpike in Elizabeth where the extensive refinery complex smelled like leaking gasoline. On several occasions, a mist was visible in the areas north and south of the refinery although it was not raining. Until the company built a sulfur scrubber, this area had its own version of acid rain. On Thanksgiving Day in 1966, an air pollution hazard event was responsible for 366 deaths in New York City.[33] Spurred on to protect the public, New Jersey made changes to the state's air pollution codes, and a rapid decline in sulfur oxides and particles followed. The state also met the U.S. National Institute for Occupational Safety and Health blood lead level standard before it was promulgated in 1978.[34]

Every medium and large city and urban places surrounded by mountains have struggled with ozone air pollution. With the proliferation of the suburbs and more cars on an expanding road network (chapter 3), photochemical smog became a chronic problem. Automobile engines have clearly improved, but with the continued increase in the number of rides, and the drift of ozone with prevailing winds that blow from the southwest to the northeast across the United States, New Jersey will not easily meet this standard.[29] Although the uptake in the use of electric vehicles may help, the increase in demand for power from generating stations may require an increase in the use of fossil fuels.

Every summer, Los Angeles, New Jersey, and states in the Northeast face ozone pollution issues. Indeed, travelers may even confront photochemical smog while driving through the bucolic farm areas of New England. Despite the persistent summer ozone problem, it would be a stretch to label New Jersey as a significant air polluter today. However, it would have been wrong to assume that air pollution was not part of the problem when the cancer atlas appeared in 1975,[3] showing high rates of lung and other respiratory cancers in New Jersey and adjacent areas of New York and Pennsylvania.

Hazardous Waste and Water Quality

Hazardous waste incidents can be spectacular. A prime example is the explosion of an illegal incinerator at the Chemical Control facility in Elizabeth, New Jersey. The explosion sent huge flames into the air, turned an adjacent river into a rainbow of colors, and sent firefighters, police, scientists, and many others on a quest to save parts of the city of Elizabeth from being destroyed. The *EPA Journal* special issue on environmental law contains an article describing the cleanup.[35] The front cover even featured a photo of the incident, showing the fireball as it rose into the night sky over the exploding drums.[36] Later that year, *Time* magazine would publish an issue with the title "The Poisoning of America."[37]

New Jersey became the poster child for hazardous waste problems, not only for the Chemical Control explosion but because the state was aggressive in identifying hazardous waste sites and seeking resources to aid in their cleanup. For example, James Florio, a former assemblyman and later the governor, became a leader in addressing the problem. Florio served as a member of the U.S. House of Representatives between 1975 in 1990 and as governor of New Jersey from January 1990 to January 1994. During his federal tenure, Florio wrote the U.S. House of Representatives version of the Comprehensive Environmental Response Compensation and Liability Act (CERCLA) of 1980, which provided a "superfund" for cleanup.

The EPA developed a preliminary list of 50,000 potential hazardous waste sites for remediation, including many in the northeast, mid-Atlantic, and Gulf Coast states, parts of California, and cities bordering the Great Lakes and the Mississippi River. The superfund initially provided sufficient resources for remediation for approximately 800 of these sites.[38]

New Jersey wanted as much money for remediation as possible to come from federal funds, so the state submitted a large portfolio of projects to remediate. Hence, EPA's initial list of 546 priority sites for cleanup included eighty-five from New Jersey. Next in rank order of the number of submissions were Michigan, Pennsylvania, New York, and Florida with forty-eight, thirty-nine, twenty-nine, and twenty-nine priority sites, respectively. Remarkably, some states, particularly in the South, submitted few sites for cleanup. New Jersey's aggressive action led to it receiving more money and receiving it earlier than other states, including money to remediate the previously described Kin-Buc Landfill. However, the state's success in obtaining funds also contributed to the notion that New Jersey was a heavily contaminated state. This fueled public concerns that cancer was directly associated with hazardous waste pollution, especially in drinking polluted water.

It is fair to say that New Jersey heavily pressured the federal government to take action to clean up hazardous waste sites; however, the state's voters supported a bond issue to begin preliminary work at these sites before federal funding was even available. The efforts to identify and remediate hazardous waste sites in New Jersey continued with governors Kean, Whitman, and McGreevy,[39] and the state strongly supported the development of better sampling tools to identify hazardous materials in the environment. Efforts to track carcinogenic materials in the environment began in New Jersey with the assistance of university scientists. The state also set up a special science group within state government to inform the governor and legislature about scientific advances in managing hazardous waste.

By the late 1980s, New Jersey and federal laws required the closing of many landfills and incinerators. The state government made a concerted effort to find safer places to manage hazardous waste within the state, but failed due to public opposition ("Not in My Backyard!"). Because of public opposition, the federal and state governments focused on pollution prevention, including replacing hazardous materials with nonhazardous ones whenever possible and recycling of hazardous materials that continued to be produced.[40,41] In 1987, state legislation mandated recycling of metal containers, glass, and many types of paper. Last on the list of pollution prevention practices was upgrading pollution controls for air, water, and land emissions.

Along with pollution prevention, New Jersey became a leading state for brownfield redevelopment. Brownfields are sites not in use or underused because of environmental contamination. With federal support, New Jersey offered funding and technical assistance for the reuse of abandoned or underused industrial and commercial sites. The state also funded research centers charged with considering creative reuses for the sites and providing technical assistance for communities with brownfield sites.[42] As a result, many former industrial sites and even some older landfills now have new uses. For instance, solar panels sprouted up on multiple closed landfills to generate electric power in 2015. We like to think that this sent a message about the importance of linking environmental protection and redevelopment.

Another way of incorporating HiAP and building a culture of health across the state is by protecting limited resources and redeveloping stressed ones. Examples include the state's regulatory authority to protect the Pinelands and the environmental and water resources in the Highlands area of New Jersey. Furthermore, heavily contaminated areas and formerly underused portions of southern Bergen County and Hudson County (e.g., Bayonne, Edgewater, Hoboken, Jersey City, Union City, Weehawken, and West New York) have been redeveloped as a "Gold Coast" that now sports highend housing and commercial development.[43] Regardless of political party, the state's elected officials and administrative staffs have made protecting the environment and the public's health into a New Jersey government ethic.

Sometimes protecting the public involves telling people what they do not want to hear. For example, Flanagan and Zhang have praised New Jersey's efforts to require private well testing, noting its importance due to the state's high population density, history of high cancer rates, and decades of dumping hazardous materials.[44] It was a major challenge for those who were tasked with informing the residents because they did not like hearing that their polluted water supply would require change. To illustrate, before telling people this bad news, the state put together a small group of professionals with risk communication experience. The group went to homes where contamination had been detected, and they spoke candidly about the problem with the homeowners. Some homeowners were aghast, and others were angry and ready to kill the messenger. Experience from these early efforts led to the development of a communication protocol for dealing with homeowners with contaminated water supplies, to direct the difficult conversations required for protecting human health.

Public Support for Environmental Protection in New Jersey

John Whitaker, a White House aide during the Nixon administration, witnessed the seeming overnight growth of public concern about environmental protection in the United States.[45] Reflecting on the first Earth Day on April 22, 1970, Whitaker emphasized that the tone of the country really changed between May 1969 and May 1971. In May 1969, only 1 percent of Americans thought that protecting the environment was important. Two years later, the number was 25 percent. Whitaker also noted that Gallup polls showed that air and water pollution as a national priority jumped from tenth to fifth place. Only war and economic issues had higher priorities. Whitaker attributed the rising concern to increasing affluence, a period of increasing activism, and a media that reinforced public concerns about the environment. Whitaker noted that the "feverish pitch" of Earth Day in 1970 later died down but did not go away. Rather, it became "part of our national ethic." This was particularly true in New Jersey.

Statewide polling data shows how strong public support for environmental protection became in New Jersey, particularly after Earth Day (Table 4.1).[46,47] A 1973 Eagleton/Star Ledger poll[46] documented how the

Table 4.1

Polling Results about Environmental Protection in New Jersey, 1973 to 2019

Question	Year (n)	Option 1 %	Option 2 %	Option 3 %	Option 4 %
Which do you consider of higher priority, encouraging or protecting the environment (ENV) or economic growth (ECON)?*	Oct. 1973 (1,235)	ENV 61	ECON 22	Don't know 17	NA
Are you in favor or opposed to easing environmental standards for business?*	Feb. 1976 (1,005)	Favor 38	Oppose 53	Don't know 9	NA
Do you think this is a very important problem, somewhat important, or not very important: protecting the environment?*	Sept. 1978 (949)	Very 66	Somewhat 29	Not very 4	Don't know 1
Over the last few years, would you say the environment in your community has become more healthy, less healthy, or stayed about the same?*	July 1986 (800)	More 8	Less 26	Same 63	Don't know 3
Overall, how serious do you think environmental problems are in New Jersey?*	March 1990 (800)	Very 61	Somewhat 30	Not too 9	Don't know 0.5
In the last 20 years, since Earth Day 1970, do you believe that environmental problems in New Jersey have gotten better, gotten worse, or stayed about the same?*	March 1990 (800)	Better 18	Worse 48	Same 28	Don't know/ depends 6
How important is protecting the environment for the next governor?*	Feb. 2004 (681)	Extremely 33	Very 41	Somewhat 22	Not at all 1

(continued)

Table 4.1
Polling Results about Environmental Protection in New Jersey, 1973 to 2019
(continued)

Question	Year (n)	Option 1 %	Option 2 %	Option 3 %	Option 4 %
To balance the state budget, some government services will be cut deeply and some will become less. Tell me if environmental programs should be cut more deeply, less deeply, or not cut at all?*	Feb. 2011 (912)	More 23	Less 43	Not at all 32	Don't know 2
Would you favor or oppose placing electricity-generating windfarms off the coast of New Jersey?**	Feb. 2019 (604)	Favor 76	Oppose 15	Don't know 10	NA
	July 2008 (496)	82	12	6	
Would you favor or oppose building another nuclear power plant in New Jersey?**	Feb. 2019 (604)	Favor 26	Oppose 67	Don't know 8	NA
	July 2008 (496)	41	51	8	
Would you favor or oppose drilling for oil or gas off the coast of New Jersey?**	Feb. 2019 (604)	Favor 30	Oppose 61	Don't know 9	NA
	July 2008 (496)	56	36	7	

Abbreviation: NA, not applicable.
SOURCES: *Eagleton Poll archive, Rutgers University.[46] **Monmouth University Polling Institute.[47]

state's residents prioritized protecting the environment over economic growth. Later, the 1976 poll showed relatively little support for weakening existing environmental standards, even though there was an economic slowdown occurring in the state.[47] The 1978 polling question showed that two-thirds of the state's respondents still continued to believe that environmental protection was a very important problem, with only 4 percent rating it not important.[48] These results were similar to the results reported for the 1990 poll.[49]

These polling questions were particularly important because they indicated that the public continued to be concerned about environmental protection, particularly in their own communities. For example, the 1986 poll question came in a time when the state had taken strong action on many environmental fronts, yet only 8 percent of respondents felt that their community environment had gotten healthier.[50] The 1990 poll found that almost half of the population thought that environmental problems had worsened. Yet between then and 1992 there was a marked increase in factory closings and a loss of manufacturing jobs, which would imply a lessening of industrial emissions.[51]

The sample polling questions from the last twenty years continued to suggest public concern, albeit perhaps not as much as during the Cancer Alley decade or during the period that followed when remediating hazardous waste sites and reducing air and water pollution were major focuses.[52,53] In New Jersey and the United States as a whole, environmental issues seem less urgent than they once were, but there remains considerable public support. For example, Monmouth University polls from 2019 show strong support for wind farms off the coast of New Jersey (see Table 4.1).[54] They also show declining support for building another nuclear power plant in the state or for drilling for gas or oil off the New Jersey coast.

In 2015 the Pew Research Center, which conducts national surveys, pulled together a series of historical questions that had asked about the trade-off between environmental standards and economic costs.[55] Their 1994 national survey had shown that 62 percent of U.S. respondents believed that "stricter environmental laws and regulations are worth the cost." By comparison, 33 percent had indicated that stricter environmental laws and regulations hurt the economy. Those results have not changed much nationally, varying between 65 percent in 2006 supporting environmental standards, to a low of 57 percent in 2013. The Pew research group asserts that increasing support for environmental protection is associated with affluence, a political leaning toward the Democrat party, and a lack of economic dependence on extractive industries. These attributes characterize the population of New Jersey.

Public Support for Cancer Protection and Control in New Jersey

We can assess public concern and support about cancer via several Eagleton/ Star Ledger polling questions of New Jersey residents (Table 4.2). Between May 1978 and in April 1985, respondents became increasingly aware of

Table 4.2
Polling Results about Cancer Prevention Programs in New Jersey, 1978 to 1995

Question	Year (n)	Option 1 %	Option 2 %	Option 3 %	Option 4 %
Do you think that people smoking in public places around you endangers your health?	May 1978 (1,004)	Yes 44	No difference 51	Don't know 5	NA
	April/ May 1985 (500)	Yes 57	No difference 40	Don't know 3	
How much money should be spent on health and hospitals?	Jan. 1979 (1,002)	More 50	Less 13	Same 34	Don't know 3
How believable is the State Department of Health about local environmental health issues?	Aug. 1987 (797)	Believable 69	Somewhat 6	Not very 22	Don't know 2
In your opinion should there or shouldn't there be insurance coverage for cancer surgery if a person is over 75 years old?	Feb. 1995 (801)	Should 84	Should not 13	Don't know 3	NA
Do you think the following is a great threat to your health?	Sept. 1995 (804)	Cancer Yes: 41	AIDS Yes: 36	Violent acts Yes: 32	Heart attack Yes: 31

Abbreviations: AIDS, acquired immunodeficiency syndrome; NA, not applicable.
SOURCE: Eagleton Poll archive, Rutgers University.[46]

secondhand smoke in public places. In January 1979, half the respondents supported more spending on health and hospitals, and only 13 percent supported less. In August 1987, the population demonstrated considerable trust in the state's Department of Health in regard to environmental health issues.

In February 1995 the public overwhelmingly supported health insurance for cancer victims. This question was perhaps the most important one of the small environmental set. In 1995 New Jersey residents were asked to rate the threat of four causes of death and morbidity. Cancer ranked first, higher than acquired immunodeficiency syndrome (AIDS), violence, and heart attacks. Governor Whitman would point to this poll response in her support for the New Jersey Commission on Cancer Research (NJCCR).

The New Jersey Commission on Cancer Research

The National Cancer Institute and the American Cancer Society (ACS) are politically powerful American organizations that have wrapped themselves around the goals of finding cures for cancer and delivering care to reduce pain and suffering. In addition to their efforts, the state of New Jersey addressed its high cancer rates in 1983 when Governor Thomas Kean created the NJCCR with a $1 million fund based on taxing cigarettes. The budget was increased to $5 million under Governor John Corzine.

Over the years, the NJCCR has provided more than $25 million for cancer research in the state. The main recipients have been young researchers as well as more seasoned ones with interesting ideas. Behind the obvious goal of reducing cancer mortality and morbidity, the NJCCR has helped build an infrastructure to help those with the disease locate cancer support services[56] as well as stimulate and incubate cancer research in the state. As Paul Wallner, former chair of the NJCCR, wrote in a letter to former Governor Jim McGreevy, "Many of our grant winners have remained in New Jersey because of their rewards. We have served as a catalyst for development of many organizational relationships for research and education, and by the development and implementation of research-related workshops, have stimulated innumerable collaborations."[57] Wallner also noted that the NJCCR has served as a model for similar programs around the country. Indeed, for every dollar that the NJCCR has awarded to grantees, the state has received an average of $4.65 in return. A more recent study showed the return even higher, at $10 returned for every dollar of investment.[58]

The NJCCR uses a rigorous procedure to obtain and evaluate grants, one similar to that used by the NCI. (We acknowledge that both authors, Michael Greenberg and Dona Schneider, have received funding from the NJCCR and used it to secure additional funds.) To gain deeper insight into the NJCCR, including the threats to its existence, we spoke with Ann Marie Hill, who was the executive director of the NJCCR for seventeen years (personal communication, June 24, 2019). Ms. Hill agreed with our assertion that the cancer atlas[2] was the trigger that led to the establishment of the NJCCR. In other words, despite the atlas's limitations, it helped the state by supporting an evidence-based response to cancer rates in New Jersey. The NJCCR has participated in multiple activities to reduce mortality and morbidity from cancer in the state and should receive at least partial credit for

- Starting a cancer registry, considered one of the better ones in the United States.
- Building up expert staff in the Departments of Health and Environmental Protection.
- Creating basic cancer research capacity in New Jersey, now estimated at over 1,000 funded scientists.
- Developing strong relationships with advocacy groups that are "unafraid to raise their voices" to government officials.
- Supporting programs on pediatric cancer.
- Leading efforts to reduce health disparities in cancer outcomes.
- Focusing on genetic screening programs.
- Supporting public health screening for breast, cervical, and prostate cancer with financial support from insurance companies (i.e., persuading them that it was in their financial and civic interests to prevent cancer deaths).
- Working with insurance companies to support clinical trials for cancer treatments.
- Working with pharmaceutical companies to develop cancer-related drugs and pilot test them in New Jersey with company funding.
- Developing and distributing approximately 100,000 copies of a cancer resource book.

Ms. Hill, now a retired professor of practice at the Edward J. Bloustein School of Planning and Public Policy at Rutgers University, sees programs such as the NJCCR as an opportunity to make decisions based on science not on misinformation or fear. She notes that several of programs that originated in New Jersey have diffused to other states and to the federal government, particularly the New Jersey Industrial Carcinogen Survey, which became the Toxic Release Inventory (TRI), and the study of psychosocial issues in former cancer patients. Part of the NJCCR's mission has included developing aids for cancer patients. She spoke proudly about the development and distribution of the *Resource Book for Cancer Patients*.[56]

The NJCCR's efforts to spur cancer research in the New Jersey had the support of both Democratic and Republican governors up to the Christie administration, which chose to eliminate or reduce the scope of both environmental and cancer research programs. Additionally, when Governor Phil Murphy removed $2 million for the NJCCR in his proposed state budget in 2018, Nicole Bodnar, an ACS Cancer Action Network volunteer, publicly criticized the move. She noted that eliminating funding for a program that "advances the fight against cancer and keeps some of the country's best researchers in the state is shortsighted."[59]

There is no question that the NCJCCR remains in jeopardy for continuing its pioneering work. The commission's work can be seen across the state with the Conquer Cancer license plates it championed. These license plates can be purchased at any time with most of the fees supporting cancer research.

Summary and Future Challenges

As the threats to the NJCCR show, sometimes creating a new and effective institution is easier than maintaining it. Here we list five challenges remaining from the Cancer Alley period that New Jersey still must address:

- Maintaining focus on a subject that seems like ancient history to many residents, most of whom will not want to hear about it again. Those who were not yet born and others who have migrated to the area since that time and are unaware of the history also must be made aware.
- Improvements in postcancer survival and reductions in dangerous exposures imply to some that the Cancer Alley problem has largely been solved. This could lead them to ignore the risks associated with indoor air quality, radon, lead in water pipes, and other related issues.
- Competition with other environmental issues such as climate change, infectious disease threats, and natural hazards may draw attention away from Cancer Alley concerns, instead of directing them toward building connections between ongoing cancer-related issues and this new generation of environmental concerns.
- New Jersey's large foreign-born population needs to be educated about cancer issues, and advocacy groups and the state need to maintain their efforts with a special focus on environmental justice–related risks.

- As healthcare costs continue to rise and the population ages, paying medical bills will increasingly take resources needed to maintain strong research on cancer-related diseases.

The Cancer Alley episode led to major investments by the state of New Jersey and helped the federal government understand the cancer challenge. It galvanized several of New Jersey's academic institutions as well as not-for-profit groups to focus on the subject. It focused the New Jersey public's attention as a whole on the issue and on its relationship with the surrounding environment. For us, this chapter offers good insight into what HiAP and a culture of health could mean.

References

1   Greenberg M. Does New Jersey cause cancer? It's how you live, not where you live, that counts. *Sciences (New York)*. 1986;26(1):40–46. doi:10.1002/j.2326-1951.1986. tb02824.x

2   Mason T, McKay F, Hoover R, et al. *Atlas of Cancer Mortality for U.S. Counties: 1950–1969*. DHEW Pub. No. (NIH) 75-780. Washington, DC: U.S. Government Printing Office; 1975.

3   Blot WJ, Fraumeni JF. Geographic patterns of bladder cancer in the United States. *JNCI J Natl Cancer Inst*. 1978;61(4):1017–1023. doi:10.1093/jnci/61.4.1017

4   Vineis P, Pirastu R. Aromatic amines and cancer. *Cancer Causes Control*. 1997; 8(3):346–355. doi:10.1023/a:1018453104303

5   Beck B. *Environmental Stewardship in a Century of Change; 1907–2007: A History of the Air and Waste Management Association's First 100 Years*. Pittsburgh: Air and Waste Management Association; 2007.

6   Woodward RL. State air pollution control activities. *Public Health Rep*. 1955; 70(5):433–436. doi:10.2307/4589095

7   State of New Jersey. Air Pollution Control Act, 1954. New Jersey Department of Environmental Protection; 1954. https://www.nj.gov/dep/enforcement/docs/air /Air%20Pollution%20Act.pdf

8   State of New Jersey. Control and Prohibition of Smoke from Combustion of Fuel; 2002. New Jersey Department of Environmental Protection. https://www.nj.gov /dep/aqm/currentrules/Sub3.pdf

9   State of New Jersey. Control and Prohibition of Open Burning; 1994. New Jersey Department of Environmental Protection. https://www.nj.gov/dep/aqm /currentrules/Sub2.pdf

10 Stern AC, ed. *Air Pollution*. 2 vols. New York: Academic Press; 1962.

11 Stern AC. Present status of atmospheric pollution in the United States. *Am J Public Health Nations Health*. 1957;47(1):78–87. doi:10.2105/ajph.47.1.78

12 Reitze AW. The legislative history of U.S. air pollution control. *Houston Law Rev*. 1999;36:679–743. https://houstonlawreview.org/api/v1/articles/4752-the -legislative-history-of-u-s-air-pollution-control.pdf

13 U.S. Environmental Protection Agency. Superfund Site: Kin-Buc Landfill, Edison Township, NJ. Updated October 20, 2017. https://cumulis.epa.gov/supercpad/cursites/csitinfo.cfm?id=0200346

14 New Jersey Legislature. New Jersey Statutes Title 26. Health and Vital Statistics 26 § 2F-2.1. https://casetext.com/statute/new-jersey-statutes/title-26-health-and-vital-statistics/chapter-262f/section-262f-21-legislative-findings-and-declaration

15 Doll R, Peto R. The causes of cancer: quantitative estimates of avoidable risks of cancer in the United States today. *J Natl Cancer Inst.* 1981;66(6):1191–1308. doi:10.1093/jnci/66.6.1192

16 Court Brown WM, Doll R. Radiation and leukæmia [letter]. *Lancet.* 1958;271(7012): 162–163. doi:10.1016/S0140-6736(58)90646-9

17 Knox JF, Holmes S, Doll R, Hill ID. Mortality from lung cancer and other causes among workers in an asbestos textile factory. *Br J Ind Med.* 1968;25(4):293–303. doi:10.1136/oem.25.4.293

18 Hamajima N, Hirose K, Tajima K, et al. Alcohol, tobacco and breast cancer—collaborative reanalysis of individual data from 53 epidemiological studies, including 58 515 women with breast cancer and 95 067 women without the disease. *Br J Cancer.* 2002;87(11):1234–1245. doi:10.1038/sj.bjc.6600596

19 Kmet J. The role of migrant population in studies of selected cancer sites: a review. *J Chronic Dis.* 1970;23(5):305–324. doi:10.1016/0021-9681(70)90015-9

20 Gordon TP, Crittenden M, Haenszel WH. End results and mortality trends in cancer. II. Cancer mortality trends in the United States, 1930–1955. *Natl Cancer Inst Monogr.* 1961;6:133–350.

21 Greenberg M, Schneider D. The cancer burden of Southern-born African Americans: analysis of a social-geographic legacy. *Milbank Q.* 1995;73(4):599. doi:10.2307/3350287

22 Greenberg MR, Schneider D, Northridge ME, Ganz ML. Region of birth and black diets: the Harlem Household Survey. *Am J Public Health.* 1998;88(8): 1199–1202. doi:10.2105/ajph.88.8.1199

23 Greenberg MR. *Urbanization and Cancer Mortality: The United States Experience, 1950–1975.* New York: Oxford University Press; 1983.

24 Centers for Disease Control and Prevention. Cancer. https://www.cdc.gov/cancer/dcpc/research/update-on-cancer-deaths/index.htm#:~:text=Is%20cancer%20increasing%20or%20decreasing,cancer%20deaths%20per%20100%2C000%20population. February 28, 2022.

25 National Cancer Institute. State Cancer Profiles. Accessed September 22, 2022. https://www.statecancerprofiles.cancer.gov/incidencerates/index.php?stateFIPS=00&areatype=state&cancer=001&race=00&sex=0&age=001&stage=999&year=0&type=incd&sortVariableName=rate&sortOrder=default&output=0#results

26 National Cancer Institute. Cancer Statistics. https://www.cancer.gov/about-cancer/understanding/statistics. Updated September 25, 2020.

27 Berman SH, Wandersman A. Fear of cancer and knowledge of cancer: a review and proposed relevance to hazardous waste sites. *Soc Sci Med.* 1990;31(1):81–90. doi:10.1016/0277-9536(90)90013-I

28 Hall B, Kerr ML. *1991–1992 Green Index: A State-by-State Guide to the Nation's Environmental Health.* Washington, DC: Island Press; 1991.

29 Lioy PJ, Georgopoulos PG. New Jersey: a case study of the reduction in urban and suburban air pollution from the 1950s to 2010. *Environ Health Perspect.* 2011; 119(10):1351–1355. doi:10.1289/ehp.1103540

30 U.S. Environmental Protection Agency. National Primary and Secondary Ambient Air Quality Standards (NAAQS) for Lead (Pb) and Implementation Plans for Lead NAAQS: 1978 Final Rule (43 FR 46246 & 46264). In: Title 40, Protection of Environment, Chapter I, Environmental Protection Agency, Subchapter C, Air Programs, Part 50, National Primary and Secondary Ambient Air Quality Standards, National Primary and Secondary Ambient Air Quality Standards for Lead. *Fed Regist.* 1978;43(194):46246–46271. https://www.epa.gov/sites/default/files/2016-03/documents/43fedreg46246.pdf

31 Stern A. Airborne particulate matter. In: *Pollution Prevention and Abatement Handbook 1998: Toward Cleaner Production.* Washington, DC: World Bank Group; 1998:201–207.

32 Wolff GT, Stroup CM, Stroup DP. The coefficient of haze as a measure of particulate elemental carbon. *J Air Pollut Control Assoc.* 2012;33(8):746–750. doi:10.1080/00022470.1983.10465635

33 Schimmel H. Evidence for possible acute health effects of ambient air pollution from time series analysis: methodological questions and some new results based on New York City daily mortality, 1963–1976. *Bull N Y Acad Med.* 1978;54(11):1052–1108. https://www.ncbi.nlm.nih.gov/pmc/articles/PMC1807672/

34 Schwemberger J, Mosby J, Doa M, et al. Blood lead levels—United States, 1999–2002. *MMWR Morb Mortal Wkly Rep.* 2005;54(20):513–516. https://www.cdc.gov/mmwr/preview/mmwrhtml/mm5420a5.htm

35 Degnan JJ, Tasher SA. Cleaning up in New Jersey. *EPA J.* 1980;6(6):10–11. https://nepis.epa.gov/Exe/ZyPDF.cgi/93000D5G.PDF?Dockey=93000D5G.PDF

36 US Environmental Protection Agency. *Environment and the Law. EPA J.* 1980;6(6). https://nepis.epa.gov/Exe/ZyPDF.cgi/93000D5G.PDF?Dockey=93000D5G.PDF

37 Magnuson E. The poisoning of America. *Time*, September 22, 1980. http://content.time.com/time/subscriber/article/0,33009,952748-1,00.html

38 Greenberg MR, Anderson RF. *Hazardous Waste Sites: The Credibility Gap.* New Brunswick, NJ: Center for Urban Policy Research; 1984.

39 Greenberg MR, Amer S. Self-interest and direct legislation: public support of a hazardous waste bond issue in New Jersey. *Polit Geogr Q.* 1989;8(1):67–78. doi:10.1016/0260-9827(89)90021-9

40 New Jersey Department of Environmental Protection. *Early Findings of the Pollution Prevention Program.* Trenton, NJ: NJDEP; 1995.

41 Freeman H. *Industrial Pollution Prevention Handbook.* New York: McGraw-Hill; 1995.

42 Greenberg M, Craighill P, Mayer H, Zukin C, Wells J. Brownfield redevelopment and affordable housing: a case study of New Jersey. *Housing Policy Debate.* 2001;12(3):515–540. doi:10.1080/10511482.2001.9521417

43 American Planning Association New Jersey Chapter. The New Jersey Gold Coast: How We Got Here and Where We Are Going [conference announcement]. October 25, 2013. https://njplanning.org/event/the-new-jersey-gold-coast-how-we-got-here-and-where-we-are-going/

44 Flanagan SV, Zheng Y. Comparative case study of legislative attempts to require private well testing in New Jersey and Maine. *Environ Sci Policy.* 2018;85:40–46. doi:10.1016/J.ENVSCI.2018.03.022

45 Whitaker JC. Earth Day recollections: what it was like when the movement took off. *EPA J.* 1988;14(6):14–17. https://nepis.epa.gov/Exe/ZyPDF.cgi/93000F5C .PDF?Dockey=93000F5C.PDF

46 Center for Public Interest Polling/Eagleton Poll, Poll #8, q138, October 1973. Eagleton Poll Archive, Rutgers University. https://eagleton.libraries.rutgers .edu/pollDetail.php?PollNum=008

47 Center for Public Interest Polling/Eagleton Poll, Poll #19, q36, February 1976. Eagleton Poll Archive, Rutgers University. https://eagleton.libraries.rutgers .edu/pollDetail.php?PollNum=019

48 Center for Public Interest Polling/Eagleton Poll, Poll #33, q28b, September 1978. Eagleton Poll Archive, Rutgers University. https://eagleton.libraries.rutgers .edu/pollDetail.php?PollNum=033

49 Center for Public Interest Polling/Eagleton Poll, Poll #78, q35, September 1990. Eagleton Poll Archive, Rutgers University. https://eagleton.libraries.rutgers .edu/pollDetail.php?PollNum=078

50 Center for Public Interest Polling/Eagleton Poll, Poll #62, q41, September 1986. Eagleton Poll Archive, Rutgers University. https://eagleton.libraries.rutgers .edu/pollDetail.php?PollNum=033

51 New Jersey Department of Labor and Workforce Development. Economic Indicators, Number 447. 2003. https://www.nj.gov/labor/labormarketinformation /tools-resources/publications-reports/economicindicators.shtml

52 Greenberg MR. Is public support for environmental protection decreasing? An analysis of U.S. and New Jersey data. *Environ Health Perspect.* 2004;112(2):121–125. doi:10.1289/ehp.6648

53 Saad L. Environmental concern down this Earth Day: economic woes may be the cause. *Gallup News Service*, April 17, 2003. https://news.gallup.com/poll/8209 /Environmental-Concern-Down-Earth-Day.aspx

54 New Jersey: strong support for wind energy. Monmouth University Polling Institute, April 3, 2019. https://www.monmouth.edu/polling-institute/reports /monmouthpoll_nj_040319/

55 Kennedy B. Public view on environment, energy and climate issues. Pew Research Center, April 18, 2018. https://www.coloradomesa.edu/energy/symposium/documents /2018presentations/5_brian_kennedy_pew_research_public_views_energy.pdf

56 Adler DL, Hill AM, New Jersey Commission on Cancer Research. *A Resource Book for Cancer Patients in New Jersey.* 6th ed. Trenton NJ: Joint Psychosocial and Nursing Advisory Group to the New Jersey Commission on Cancer Research; 2007.

57 Wallner P. New Jersey Commission on Cancer Research 2002 Annual Report. Trenton, NJ; 2002.

58 New Jersey Commission on Cancer Research. 2018–19 Annual Report. February 4, 2021. https://www.nj.gov/health/ces/cancer-researchers/njccr/NJCCR%20 Annual%20Report%202020.pdf

59 Bodnar N. Letter: Murphy should restore cancer research funds. [New Jersey] *Courier-Post*. April 29, 2018. https://www.courierpostonline.com/story/opinion /readers/2018/04/29/governor-phil-murphy-should-restore-new-jersey -commission-cancer-research-funds/562880002/

5

Health Disparities and the COVID-19 Pandemic

―――――――――――――――――――――――――――●

"A riot is the language of the unheard."
—Martin Luther King Jr.[1]

Riots, unlawful behaviors, and peaceful protests are public expressions of frustration that were apparent during the last half century. Examples include the civil rights movements of the 1960s; the antiwar marches and the rise in domestic terror groups of the 1970s; the rise in gun violence, civil unrest, and crack epidemic in the 1980s; and the continued efforts of women, gays and lesbians, and African Americans who organized many thousands to march for their rights over the past decades. These openly public expressions are visible to anyone with a mass media connection, but this chapter focuses instead on the mostly silent expressions of pain associated with disparities that few of us ever see—those associated with health.

Unrelenting segregation and grinding poverty contribute to health disparities directly through differences in exposures as well as in access to prevention and treatments. They also contribute indirectly through differences in education, housing, and other opportunities and services that people need to be healthy. This chapter has four objectives:

1   Examine health disparities and health-risk factors among New Jersey's racial/ethnic groups and in its poorest cities before and during the COVID-19 pandemic.

2   Examine health disparities in the United States and in New Jersey's poorest cities as demonstrated by COVID-19 pandemic.

3   Review cascading effects associated with health disparities for youth and the economy.

4   Consider the challenges underscored by the pandemic and the roles of government and residents of New Jersey in addressing them.

Health Disparities in New Jersey before the Pandemic

The starting point for examining health disparities is by obtaining mortality rates for different places by race and gender, adjusted for age differences. Adjustment for age is essential because the probability of dying increases with age, especially after sixty-five years. For example, Alaska and Utah have the lowest crude death rates among all the states, but this is explained by the low proportion of their populations aged sixty-five years and older (<12 percent). By contrast, over 20 percent of the populations in Florida and Maine are sixty-five years and older. Thus, these two states have much higher crude death rates than Alaska and Utah.[2]

The New Jersey Department of Health collects a massive amount of data that demonstrates both health disparities and the conditions that lead to them. Table 5.1 shows New Jersey's age-adjusted mortality rates for 2017–2019 (before the pandemic) and the provisional 2020 rates (after the pandemic struck).[3] Most striking are the low age-adjusted death rates for Asian residents in the state in both time periods. Equally apparent are the high rates for New Jersey's non-Hispanic Blacks (39 percent higher than the state rate and more than double that of Asian residents), again in both time periods. Note that every racial/ethnic combination had a much higher rate in 2020 than in the three prior years, explained by the fact that COVID-19 cases are included in the latter rates. The "smallest" increase in rates between the two time periods was for non-Hispanic whites (15 percent). The increase for non-Hispanic Blacks added to the highest rates for this group in both time periods. The increases for both non-Hispanic Asians and Hispanics were higher than for non-Hispanic Blacks, at 58 and 72 percent,

Table 5.1

Age-Adjusted Death Rates per 100,000 for New Jersey, with Numbers of Deaths and Estimated Populations, 2020

Racial/Ethnic Group	Number of Deaths, 2020	Estimated Population, 2020	Age-Adjusted Death Rate, 2017–2019*	Age-Adjusted Death Rate, 2020*
Non-Hispanic Black	13,668	1,148,564	828.4	1152.5
Non-Hispanic white	65,333	4,850,995	701.2	807.9
Non-Hispanic Asian	3,798	870,472	301.8	477.4
Hispanic (all races)	10,852	1,856,844	463.2	797.1
Total**	95,637	8,882,190	661.5	837.2

*Calculated on the U.S. 2000 population standard.
**Includes cases with no and multiple racial/ethnic designations.
SOURCE: New Jersey Department of Health.[3]

respectively. We have never seen anything like these increases in death rates except in countries ravaged by war. The virus inflicted death and morbidity similar to that which we would expect from bombs, bullets, starvation, and other deprivations associated with major conflicts.

Death rates present stark evidence of health disparities. However, the state's Behavioral Risk Factor Survey (NJBRFS)[4] and ongoing data collection systems[5] also allow us to compare health-risk indicators for New Jersey residents during the prepandemic period. Table 5.2 presents the percentages of the state's non-Hispanic Black, non-Hispanic White, and Hispanic residents for each of the indicators, with symbols to signal whether it is statistically significantly higher (+), similar to (=), or worse than (−) that for New Jersey as a whole. The data show that non-Hispanic whites had eight indicators considered better than the state's; ten were similar, and only one was lower. The clear advantage for non-Hispanic whites was in the indicators related to health care access. By contrast, non-Hispanic Blacks had lower percentages compared with the state as a whole in eight categories; Hispanics had lower ones in five. Of note are the low percentages of non-Hispanic Blacks and Hispanics receiving vaccines for pneumonia and influenza, along with less health insurance coverage and high rates of obesity, which were precursors for bad COVID-19 outcomes.

Although the data in Table 5.2 show clear distinctions in health-risk indicators by race and ethnicity, we must point out that income is not explicitly part of these data. Some countries automatically collect and integrate

Table 5.2

Percentages of Health-Risk Indicators for Racial/Ethnic Populations in New Jersey with Comparisons to the State as a Whole

Health-Risk Indicator (Data Year)	Non-Hispanic Black %	Non-Hispanic White %	Hispanic (All Races) %
Lack of health insurance coverage (2018)	9.2 (=)	5.0 (+)	18.5 (−)
Consume 1+ soda per day in past 7 days (2019)	16.5 (−)	9.0 (=)	9.5 (=)
Women			
No prenatal care (2017)	3.9 (−)	1.0 (+)	1.5 (=)
First trimester prenatal care (2018)	58.5 (−)	81.3 (+)	65.6 (−)
Alcohol use during last 3 months of pregnancy (2018)	4.3 (+)	12.3 (=)	8.7 (=)
Low-risk cesarean deliveries (2018)	31.5 (−)	26.5 (+)	27.7 (=)
Vaginal birth after previous cesarean delivery (2017)	10.9 (=)	13.9 (+)	10.0 (−)
Safe sleep, mothers, infants on their back to sleep (2018)	62.6 (−)	85.7 (+)	58.2 (−)
Age 21–65 who had Pap test during the last 3 years (2017)	81.6 (=)	85.1 (=)	84.0 (=)
Age 50–74 who had mammogram in past 2 years (2017)	80.2 (=)	78.3 (=)	87.9 (+)
Men			
Age 40+ years who talked with health professional about prostate-specific antigen test (2015)	34.7 (+)	22.9 (=)	22.7 (=)
Adults			
Always wore seat belts in automobiles (2017)	88.2 (=)	90.6 (=)	88.9 (=)
Reported cigarette smoking (2017)	15.3 (=)	15.9 (=)	13.3 (=)
Influenza vaccination in past 12 months, age 65+ (2017)	57.7 (=)	64.5 (=)	64.6 (=)
Ever received pneumococcal vaccination (2017)	63.6 (−)	75.5 (+)	51.6 (−)
Physically active 65+ years (2017)	49.7 (−)	64.4 (=)	54.2 (=)
Reporting sunburn in past year (2015)	5.0 (+)	26.6 (−)	11.4 (+)
Adolescents			
Participating in physical activity, 60+ minutes, 5+ days a week (2019)	31.3 (=)	49.9 (+)	45.9 (=)
Video/computer game time grades 9–12 (2019)	55.7 (=)	53.6 (=)	52.8 (=)

Key: Statistically significantly higher (+), similar to (=), or worse than (−) that for New Jersey as a whole ($P < 0.05$).
SOURCE: New Jersey Department of Health.[4,5]

socioeconomic status data into their health outcomes data, but the United States does not. Thus, the health-risk indicators may underestimate actual health disparities.

Joint Effects of Race/Ethnicity and Socioeconomic Status

As a surrogate for the joint effects of race/ethnicity and income, we selected six New Jersey cities marked by high concentrations of poor and minority populations. Atlantic City, Camden, Newark, Passaic, Paterson, and Trenton have long been home to a large proportion of these residents. For example, in 1959 all six of these cities had families with a median household income of less than $3,000. In 1960, all six had 11 percent or more of their population with less than five years of school attendance. In 1960, what the U.S. Census labeled "minority" proportions exceeded 15 percent in few New Jersey cities; however, among these six cities, Newark had the highest proportion at 34 percent, and only Passaic did not pass the 15 percent threshold.[6]

Six decades later, this long-established pattern of poor and minority populations in the selected cities persists—arguably it has intensified. Because Atlantic City has the smallest population, and as the state calculates age-adjusted death rates only for cities of 65,000 or more people, we reluctantly had to eliminate it from our city comparisons in Table 5.3. Hence, the table compares the age-adjusted death rates for five New Jersey cities, and for the racial/ethnic combinations for the state as a whole in 2020.[7] We note that each city had a higher age-adjusted death rate than did any single race/ethnic combination, indicating the importance of including socioeconomic variables when examining health disparities.

Table 5.4 provides more information about the concentration of poor and minority populations in the six New Jersey cities. Five of the twenty-five metrics in Table 5.4 are about demographics, six measure the indoor and outdoor community environments, and fourteen measure health outcomes and services. The data are from multiple sources; to simplify the presentation, we prepared a six city aggregate by weighting the city data by population size. We were not able to include Atlantic City in twelve of the fourteen health-related comparisons, and these are designated by asterisks in the table. Four of the environmental comparisons assume the overall average for the state to be 50 percent, and these are denoted by a hash sign.

Beginning with population size, in 1960, 891,000 people (14.7 percent of the state population) lived in the six cities. By 2019, the population of

Table 5.3

Age-Adjusted Death Rates per 100,000 for Cities and Racial/Ethnic Groups, New Jersey, 2020

Place or Population	Age-Adjusted Death Rate per 100,000*
City	
Camden	1,318.0
Newark	1,186.4
Passaic	1,193.8
Paterson	1,171.8
Trenton	1,227.0
Racial/ethnic group, NJ	
Non-Hispanic Black	1,152.5
Non-Hispanic white	807.9
Non-Hispanic Asian	477.4
Hispanic (all races)	797.1
Total	837.2

NOTE: Calculated on the U.S. 2000 population standard.
SOURCE: New Jersey Department of Health.[7]

these cities was only 691,000 (7.8 percent of the state population). With the exception of Atlantic City, which is a tourist center, the other five cities lost their status as major manufacturing centers and became places with much smaller economies. They have five times as many African American and six times as many Latino residents as the state as a whole; 89 percent of their populations fit the definition of "people of color" as defined by President Clinton's 1994 presidential executive order on environmental justice.[16] The poverty rate for the six cities is almost four times that for the state as a whole.

The collective local environments for the six cities are challenging. For example, the attorney general's office collects information about guns found at crime scenes.[10] With less than 8 percent of the state's population, these six cities reported almost 34 percent of the guns recovered at crimes during the period March 2020 to March 2021. Furthermore, the number of guns collected at crimes increased by 50 percent between September 2020 and March 2021.

The recovered guns data are consistent with several other distressing trends. One is the spread of the opioid epidemic. Drake et al.[17] estimated nearly 400,000 deaths in the United States from opioids from 1999 through 2017. New Jersey ranked number 10 in the opioid-related death rate.[18] County-scale data show a disproportionate number of cases in southern

Table 5.4

Summary Metrics for Six New Jersey Cites (Atlantic City, Camden, Newark, Passaic, Paterson, and Trenton) Compared with New Jersey as a Whole

Metric	Six Cities (Ratio to State)
Demographic	
Population, % of NJ residents in six cities, 2019[8]	7.8 (NA)
African American/Black, % living in six cities, 2019[8]	39.0 (5.00)
Latino-Hispanic, % living in six cities, 2019[8]	46.8 (6.00)
Poverty, % living in poverty in six cities, 2019[8,9]	30.6 (3.92)
Unemployment rate, 2019[8]	13.4 (1.74)
Environmental	
Guns confiscated in crimes, % in six cities, March 2020–March 2021[10]	33.9 (4.34)
Local fair share per student from city budget, 2017 compared with state weighted average[11]	$3,219 (0.23)
Indoor lead exposure (as % pre-1960 housing) in six cities compared with all state areas[12,13]	69 (1.38)#
Particles 2.5 ppm, % in six cites compared to all state areas[12,13]	67 (1.34)#
Traffic proximity, % in six cities compared to all state areas[12,13]	84 (1.68)#
Hazardous waste proximity, % in six cities compared to all state areas[12,13]	78 (1.56)#
Health-Related	
Infant mortality rate for the six cities, 2014–2018 (deaths per 1,000 births)[5]	8.2 (1.91)
HIV/AIDS deaths, % living in six cities, cumulative thru December 31, 2018[14]	35.7 (4.57)
Binge drinking, age-adjusted prevalence rate among adults, 2014–2016[15*]	13.7 (0.81)
Smoking, age-adjusted prevalence rate among adults, 2014–2016[15*]	23.8 (1.53)
Obesity, age-adjusted prevalence rate among adults, 2014–2016[15*]	38.1 (1.43)
Asthma, age-adjusted prevalence rate among adults, 2014–2016[15*]	10.7 (1.29)
Cancer, age-adjusted prevalence rate among adults, 2014–2016[15*]	4.5 (0.87)
Diagnosed diabetes, age-adjusted prevalence rate among adults, 2014–2016[15*]	15.6 (1.80)
Mental health not good for >14 days during the last month among adults, 2014–2016[15*]	15.8 (1.49)
Physical health not good for >14 days during the last month among adults, 2014–2016[15*]	17.8 (1.82)
Lack of health insurance for those 18–64 years old, 2014–2016[15*]	31.0 (1.97)
Mammography among women 50–74 years old, 2014–2016[15*]	74.2 (0.94)
Pap smear among women 21–65 years old, 2014–2016[15*]	75.6 (0.90)
Fecal occult blood test, sigmoidoscopy, or colonoscopy among those 50–75 years old, 2014–2016[15*]	50.9 (0.81)

Abbreviations: AIDS, acquire immunodeficiency syndrome; HIV, human immunodeficiency virus; NA, not available; ppm, parts per million.

SOURCE: U.S. Census Bureau,[8] Raychaudhuri (2019),[9] New Jersey State Police,[10] *New Jersey Education Aid* (2017),[11] U.S. Environmental Protection Agency (2021),[12,13] New Jersey Department of Health,[14] Centers for Disease Control and Prevention (2020).[15]

*Data do not include Atlantic City.

#The average for the state is 50%.

New Jersey, a fact consistent with the higher rates of opioid use among rural and suburban non-Hispanic whites.[19,20] The Advocacy Resource Center of the American Medical Association[21] summarized its concern about the increase in opioid use related to the COVID-19 pandemic. Both Drake et al.[17] and the Substance Abuse and Mental Health Administration[21,22] noted a rapid increase among minorities living in cities. Thus, although the opioid epidemic has been linked to rural and suburban non-Hispanic Whites, the problem has been spreading to minority populations as well. The Partners for Women and Justice Center at the Seton Hall Law School[23] reported another disconcerting trend: COVID-19 has intensified domestic violence in New Jersey.

Two indicators in Table 5.4 focus on schools and housing-related hazards. The table includes the estimated local fair share per student from city budgets in 2017 compared with the state weighted average. The weighted school district average ratio for the Abbott districts (designation for five of the cities) was 0.23—in other words, less than one-fourth of the state average. Notably, Atlantic City was not one of the original Abbott school districts because of the considerable casino-generated revenues at that time. However, the casinos have been closing, and Atlantic City would now qualify as an Abbott district based on lack of local revenue. (See chapter 6 for more about the New Jersey Supreme Court's *Abbott* school case.)

Chapter 6 offers compelling evidence of the relationship between poor quality housing and public health. Lead exposure is among the most serious problems for children younger than six years because it can severely affect their mental and physical development. The U.S. Environmental Protection Agency (EPA) has estimated that between 1927 and 1987, 68 million American children were exposed to toxic levels of lead from leaded gasoline alone.[24] Although the 1996 ban on the use of leaded gasoline for on-road vehicles helped reduce lead exposure, cities with much of their housing stock built before 1960 continue to expose children to lead through old paint, dust, and soil exposures. Table 5.4 offers metrics from the EPA's EJScreen database.[12,13] One of these is based on proportion of homes built before 1960, the time when lead paint was rapidly declining in the in-home environment. The six cities were listed as having 69 percent of their housing stock built before 1960, 1.38 times higher than the state average at 50 percent. In other words, in-home exposure to lead in these six cities is 38 percent more likely than elsewhere in New Jersey.

The six cities are also more likely to pose health risks from exposures to fine particles (2.5 ppm), auto and truck traffic, and potentially to effluent and accidents from hazardous waste sites (67, 84, and 78 percent, respectively). The particulate data come from air quality monitoring stations, whereas the traffic and hazardous waste metrics are derived by measuring the distance from the centroid of the city to the nearest major highways and hazardous waste sites. In other words, the outdoor environmental metrics as well as that for the indoor lead are unfavorable in the six cities compared with all the jurisdictions in the state.

The overall picture for health metrics in the six cities is similarly distressing. Infant mortality, one of the world's most widely used indicators, shows the six-city rate is almost double that for the state as a whole.[5] Similarly, although the six cities have less than 8 percent of the state's population, they have more than one-third of the state's cumulative human immunodeficiency virus/acquire immunodeficiency syndrome (HIV/AIDS) deaths. A brighter metric is that binge drinking among adults is less in the six cities than the state as a whole. However, rates for smoking, obesity, and asthma are higher, as they are for mental and physical health-related stresses for the month when people were surveyed.

Table 5.4 shows that access to health care in the six cities is problematic, as demonstrated by the relative lack of health insurance among those younger than sixty-five years old. Access to prevention is also of concern: mammographies (94 percent), Pap smears (90 percent), and colon tests (81 percent) are less prevalent in the six cities, after adjusting for age. Overall and with few exceptions the data provide clear evidence of health disparities in the six cities compared with the state as a whole. These disparities, characterized by a great deal of poverty, are located in cities primarily inhabited by people of color.

Health Disparities Demonstrated by the COVID-19 Pandemic

A rapidly growing literature tried to keep pace with the spread of COVID-19 and its impacts. The Centers for Disease Control and Prevention (CDC) began continuously monitoring COVID-19–related disparities at the beginning of the pandemic. Their December 2020 summary report[25] showed marked disparities by race/ethnicity. Researchers quickly focused on spread of the virus and disease during the first 3 to 4 months (the first wave), which lasted through June 2020. Finch and Finch[26] used CDC county-scale data for 2,853 of the nation's 3,007 counties for seventy-one days from late January 2020 through early April 2020—in other words, very early in the U.S. pandemic. Urban counties with high poverty indexes had many more confirmed cases than others. Deaths followed with roughly a two-week lag. The authors found that poor people living in large cities could not stay home: they had to travel to work by mass transit and were less able to practice social distancing. By April 2020, however, Finch and Finch found that cases had spread to the more affluent areas. As the disease spread, resources for testing were shifted to the more affluent areas, even though the numbers of cases remained higher in poorer neighborhoods.

Brown and Ravallion[27] also used U.S. county-scale data and found a strong relationship between deaths, poverty, race/ethnicity, density, and, of course, age. Notably, they observed both separate and connected poverty- and race/ethnicity-related disparities in COVID-19 outcomes. The researchers added two interesting observations. The first was that although poor and disadvantaged minorities bore the brunt of the impact, it was the more affluent who were stressed by needing to adjust to new home and workplace conditions that many found overwhelming. The elderly, many of whom were retired and able to socially distance, had pre-existing conditions that compounded their risks. This led to extremely high mortality for this group, most notably for those residing in nursing homes.

Abedi et al.[28] focused on 369 counties in seven states with the most COVID-19 infections through April 9, 2020: California, Louisiana, Massachusetts, Michigan, New York, New Jersey, and Pennsylvania. Populous counties with diverse populations, including those with higher incomes and education levels, were at higher risk of infections. However, deaths were more likely in the less populated counties with higher disability and poverty rates.

Kabarriti et al.[29] analyzed information gathered about 5,902 patients who came to Montefiore Hospital in the Bronx, New York during the period March 14 through April 15, 2020. This was in the early stages of the epidemic, but the Bronx already had the highest COVID-19 infection rates in New York City, which had the highest rates in the United States. Some of the research team's observations were anticipated. Risk increased markedly after age sixty, and especially after age eighty. Obesity, dementia, and kidney disease were strong predictors of death. Non-Hispanic Blacks and Hispanic patients were more likely to have multiple comorbidities and test positive for COVID-19. After controlling for age, sex, and comorbidities, survival rates were similar to those for non-Hispanic Whites, which the authors could not explain.

The virus continued to spread during the summer of 2020. Seligman et al.[30] studied the correlates of the first 200,000 reported U.S. deaths through September 2020. They reported the odds of dying from COVID-19 were 2.56 for Hispanics and 3.68 for African Americans compared to non-Hispanic Whites. The major marker used for predicting socioeconomic status was education. Those with less than a high school education had the greatest chance of death. In contrast, those with a four-year college degree or higher had an odds ratio of 0.90. In other words, higher educational achievement was protective (see also Bialek et al.[31] for geographic differences in COVID-19 outcomes; Roxby et al.[32] for virus detection and COVID-19-related outcomes for older adults; and Garg et al.[33] for characteristics of patients hospitalized with COVID-19.)

Doti[34] stepped back from hospital and county-scale analyses to examine state data for policies on health outcomes from the pandemic. He argued that states play a pivotal role in federalist political systems like the United States, and hence interstate differences are important. Using regression analysis, Doti observed an association with population density and poverty (not median family income and other standard income measures). He did not find an association with race/ethnicity at the state scale. The contribution of this study was to divide the year 2020 into two periods and examine the impact of the Oxford stringency index on death rates. The index includes policy measures such as closing schools and workplaces, reducing transit, canceling public events, placing restrictions on public gatherings, requiring people to stay at home, administering contact tracing, COVID-19 testing policy, and more. He concluded that population density was the strongest correlate of COVID-19 death rates during the first half of the year but not a significant predictor in the second half of the year. His point was that stringent policy actions lowered death rates.

To summarize, researchers used information aggregated by counties, states, and medical institutions to understand the destructive path that the COVID-19 virus followed from Wuhan to the United States. The virus spread relatively quickly in New Jersey. The state is one of the world's most accessible urban corridors, served by multiple airports and trains, and marked by high-density living and working conditions. These assets have brought great wealth to New Jersey but also increased the population's risk for spreading COVID-19. Without a good understanding of the diffusion variables, it took time to learn that people were at high risk because of pre-existing health conditions, age-related immunological deficiencies, and the inability to social distance because of the need to work and interact as part of their routine lives. Additionally, many had limited access to medical care and COVID-19 testing opportunities. Poverty and race/ethnicity, as they do in education, housing, and so many other parts of life, were quickly woven into the COVID-19 fabric.

Health Disparities Related to COVID-19 in New Jersey

Chapter 2 summarized the overall impact of COVID-19 and Table 5.1 compared the age-adjusted death rates for New Jersey before the pandemic and in 2020. Using the state's counts, Table 5.5 summarizes the COVID-19 effect on mortality in New Jersey. It enumerates both racial/ethnic disparities across the state and socioeconomic factors as represented by the six cities. We used the *International Classification of Diseases, Tenth Revision* (ICD-10), code U07.1 to identify deaths, which is the COVID-19 cause now used on all U.S. death certificates.[35] This code does not include other deaths that might have been hastened by COVID-19.

With these caveats noted, two patterns stand out in Table 5.5. First is the remarkably high COVID-19 death rates for Hispanic and non-Hispanic Black New Jersey residents in 2020. Their rates were more than twice those for non-Hispanic whites. Second is the high COVID-19 age-adjusted death rates for the cities of Paterson and Passaic. These results are related to the racial/ethnic characteristics: Passaic's population is over 75 percent Hispanic, and Paterson's is over 60 percent. These cities host a higher proportion of Hispanic residents than do Camden, Newark, Trenton, and the state as a whole.

The racial/ethnic and spatial disparities in mortality from COVID-19 in 2020 shown in Table 5.5 are even more striking when examined by age group. Table 5.6 shows that non-Hispanic whites had relatively low rates of COVID-19 mortality before age sixty-five years, but then the risk increases in age groups sixty-five to seventy-four years, seventy-five to eighty-four years,

Table 5.5

COVID-19–Related Deaths and Age-Adjusted Death Rates, New Jersey Cities and Racial/Ethnic Populations, 2020

Place or Population	Number of COVID-19 Deaths*	COVID-19 Age-Adjusted Death Rate*	All Causes, Age-Adjusted Death Rate
City			
Atlantic City	49	NA	NA
Camden	114	178.6	1,318.0
Newark	744	297.4	1,186.4
Passaic	246	457.8	1,193.8
Paterson	443	343.6	1,171.8
Trenton	186	229.4	1,227.0
Total six	1,782	NA	NA
Racial/Ethnic Group, New Jersey			
Non-Hispanic Black	2,557	215.7	1,152.5
Non-Hispanic white	8,838	104.1	807.9
Non-Hispanic Asian	951	117.7	477.4
Hispanic (all races)	3,519	256.1	797.1
Total**	16,388	141.8	837.2

NOTE: Calculated on the U.S. 2000 population standard. NA indicates data not available.
*International Classification of Diseases, Tenth Revision (ICD-10), code U07.1.
**Includes cases with no and multiple racial/ethnic designations.
SOURCE: New Jersey Department of Health.[3]

Table 5.6

Age-Specific Death Rates per 100,000 for COVID-19 with Ratios Comparing Racial/Ethnic Group Rate to the State Rate, New Jersey, 2020

Age group in Years	Number of COVID-19 Deaths	Age-Specific Death Rates from COVID-19	Ratio of Non-Hispanic Black Rate to State Rate	Ratio of Non-Hispanic White Rate to State Rate	Ratio of Non-Hispanic Asian Rate to State Rate	Ratio of Hispanic (All Races) Rate to State Rate
25–34	116	10.1	1.83	NA	NA	2.07
35–44	299	26.3	1.40	0.33	NA	2.33
45–54	879	73.2	1.67	0.35	0.52	2.36
55–64	2,148	175.5	1.74	0.52	0.81	2.37
65–74	3,341	401.1	1.82	0.66	0.92	2.10
75–84	4,332	985.5	1.60	0.79	0.83	1.76
85+	5,256	2,587.8	1.12	0.95	0.93	1.24

NOTE: Calculated on the U.S. 2000 population standard. Some racial/ethnic rates are based on few cases, and the 2020 numbers are provisional. NA indicates data not available.
SOURCE: NJ Department of Health.[3]

and eighty-four years and older. Despite this increase, the ratio to the state as a whole never exceeded 1. By strong contrast, the Hispanic rates were more than double the state rates by age twenty-five to thirty-four years, and they remained so through age group sixty-five to seventy-four years. The rates then dropped below 2.0 but remained elevated. The non-Hispanic Black rates followed the Hispanic pattern.

Overall, with the caveat that the 2020 data we used for the analysis were provisional and may slightly change when finalized, we identified substantial health disparities associated with COVID-19 for the state's Hispanic and non-Hispanic Black populations. The disparities were particularly marked in the state's poor cities with high levels of poverty and minorities.

Chasing Herd Immunity

Herd immunity is a stage in an infectious disease process when the population as a whole is protected because a sufficient proportion of is no longer susceptible. This is because many have already had the disease and are immune or because they have been successfully immunized. We now know, for example, that to prevent measles epidemics about 95 percent of a population needs to be vaccinated. For polio, the herd immunity threshold is about 80 percent; for influenza it is about 50 percent.[36] Unfortunately, when COVID-19 emerged, there was no definitive knowledge of the level of herd immunity that must be achieved or how long it must be maintained in order to curb the pandemic. Without that knowledge and without a vaccine, it was important to encourage people to be proactive with hand washing, using personal protective equipment such as masks, and social distancing. Early estimates were that the threshold to achieve herd immunity for severe acute respiratory syndrome coronavirus 2 (SARS-CoV-2, or COVID-19) would be between 60 and 70 percent, which seemed potentially achievable once vaccines became available.[37]

Assuming the goal is for at least 70 percent of the population to be fully vaccinated, as of late May 2021 New Jersey had a long way to go (46 percent fully vaccinated; 58 percent with one dose); the United States as a whole had an even a longer path (39 percent fully vaccinated; 49 percent with one dose).[38] New Jersey ranked seventh among the fifty states in the proportion of its residents who received the vaccine.[39] Seven of the ten states with over 40 percent fully vaccinated were in the Northeast (Connecticut, Maine,

Massachusetts, New Jersey, New York, Rhode Island, and Vermont). New Mexico, Hawaii, and South Dakota were the remaining three.

It took time and a great deal of effort for New Jersey to reach an immunization rate of even 40 percent. On March 15, 2021, the Associated Press[40] reported that New Jersey had reached a million fully vaccinated and 3 million residents with at least one shot. In March 2021, Governor Phil Murphy expanded eligibility to teachers and other school staff, transportation workers, the homeless, tribal communities, migrant farm workers, and childcare employees. On that date, 11.4 percent of the national population was fully vaccinated, while in New Jersey 12.2 percent were. Murphy's stated goal was to reach 70 percent by June 2021. In late April 2021, Conway et al.[41] reported that enough vaccine would be available to vaccinate every eligible adult in the United States by the end of May 2021. But consumer demand was declining. Conway et al. argued for "prioritize[ing] equity," asserting that rural communities had the highest death rates followed by Black communities. They recommend enhancing scheduling systems, offering vaccinations at employment sites, and providing support for those who need time off to be vaccinated. By mid-2022, vaccinations of New Jerseyans sixty-four years of age and older approached 95 percent; those 12 to 17 years were at about 60 percent; and those aged 5 to 11 years were about 30 percent. About three out of ten of children aged five to eleven years were vaccinated. Vaccinations for the youngest proceeded more slowly.

Ndugga et al.[42] discussed race/ethnicity vaccination rates compared to population size, cases and deaths at the state scale. On May 3, 2021, CDC reported that race/ethnicity was known for 55 percent of the people who received at least one dose, of whom 66 percent were white, 13 percent Hispanic, 9 percent Black, and 6 percent Asian. Others reporting were American Indians, Alaskan natives, native Hawaiians, and multiple race pairings. Nationally, Ndugga et al.[42] reported that Black and Hispanic people received smaller proportions of COVID-19 immunizations compared with their numbers of cases, deaths, and population size. In New Jersey, whites had 60 percent of COVID-19 immunizations compared with 47 percent of the cases, 57 percent of the deaths, and 54 percent of the population. Asians also received a larger share of COVID-19 vaccinations (11 percent) compared with their number of cases (5 percent), deaths (6 percent), and population size (11 percent). The state's Black residents received 7 percent of the COVID-19 vaccinations compared with their constituting 12 percent of the cases,

16 percent of the deaths, and 12 percent of the population. Among Hispanics, 12 percent received vaccines while they represented 17 percent of the cases, 21 percent of the deaths, and 21 percent of the population. We remind the reader that these data are partial and comparisons are undermined by missing data. Nevertheless, they show alarming health disparities by race and ethnicity for Blacks and Hispanics early in the epidemic, which is our emphasis and continues below.

As this chapter was written, data for New Jersey cities was available only to the public in not easily readable maps. On May 3, 2021, Mueller[43] reported that the governor's office listed sixteen municipalities of 10,000+ persons where less than 40 percent of their eligible residents had received at least one dose of the vaccine. Included on that list were Camden (32 percent), Trenton (32 percent), Newark (38 percent), and Passaic (39 percent), four of the six cities used to demonstrate health disparities in this chapter. All sixteen places listed by the governor's office as underimmunized were low-income municipalities, ranking between 595 and 702 on a list of ranked per capita income for the 702 places in New Jersey. The publication of the governor's list led to increased vaccinations in some of these places.[44]

The governor was quoted as stating that "this mapping tool is not meant to create competitions among communities, nor is it meant to shame any communities." As part of the push toward vaccination, the governor authorized the Pfizer vaccine for ages twelve to fifteen years, redeployed resources to places with low vaccination rates, and considered paying for vaccine-hesitant people to be vaccinated,[45] many of whom are less than trusting of authorities.

As the pandemic moved beyond the first year, doubts arose as to whether herd immunity could be achieved for the disease. Independent data scientist Youyang Gu developed a disease forecasting model for COVID-19 that he called "Path to Herd Immunity." In February 2021, Gu changed the name of the model to "Path to Normality," noting that reaching the herd immunity threshold was unlikely because of vaccine hesitancy, the emergence of new variants, and the delayed arrival of vaccinations for children.[46] Aschwanden[37] agreed, listing five reasons why herd immunity might not be attainable:

1 It is unclear whether vaccines prevent transmission.
2 The vaccine rollout was uneven.
3 New variants change the herd immunity equation.

4 Immunity might not last forever.
5 Vaccines might change human behavior.

A return to normality with COVID-19 and its variants as an endemic disease became a more realistic goal than achieving herd immunity. Although the new vaccines and vaccine programs did reduce hospitalizations and deaths from COVID-19, they could not eradicate the disease and its variants. The ability to vaccinate the willing as well as our most vulnerable, along with the ability to provide screening and early treatment at home, has been effective in allowing a return to school and work—providing a semblance of normality.

Cascading Effects on Youth and the Economy

The health disparities observed in this chapter understate the impact of COVID-19 because the disease's effects cascade through other systems, not only health but also education, housing, and the economy. These effects compound the accumulated decades of grinding poverty, segregation, substandard housing, redlining, and lack of educational opportunity for a not-insignificant proportion of the U.S. population. We briefly highlight several major challenges, beginning with those facing American youth.

The immediate and long-term impacts of the pandemic on children and young adults are of serious concern, particularly in the areas of education and socialization. Most public schools and many private schools as well as preschools and day care centers closed during the pandemic. Asserting that 80 percent of the world's children were closed out of schools, Van Lancker and Parolin[47] characterized these COVID-19 closures as a "social crisis in the making." Without school, some parents had to give up their jobs to care for their children. Education continued but was drastically altered, especially among those who had little or no access to computers and teachers. At this time, we have no data about educational performance other than what we have observed among our own college students, who were unable or barely able to cope when they had to transition to online learning modes mid-semester. In the first year of the pandemic, we saw far more withdrawals, incompletes, and low grades than at any time in our experience. We can only surmise that the income and race/ethnicity educational gap also grew among younger children.

Haseltine[48] described COVID-19 as a "systematic shock to the determinants of child health, affecting family functioning and income. When schools closed, some children lost one nutritious meal a day, . . . as well as access to health care and education" (2). This was a tragedy; Schwartz and Rothbart[49] had reported the positive impact of extending free school lunch to all students, regardless of income, on academic performance in New York City middle schools. They found the program increased academic performance by as much as 0.083 standard deviations in math and 0.059 in English language arts for nonpoor students; smaller but still statistically significant effects of 0.032 and 0.027 standard deviations were found in math and English language arts for poor students. There was also some evidence that participation in school lunch improved weight outcomes for nonpoor students.

The impact of the pandemic on housing was multidimensional. People living in crowded conditions were at home more than they had previously been. Their electricity, water, and other utility bills increased, and their homes might not have been able to handle the increased demand for internet and appliance use. In some households, children had to share computers or compete with each other for online class time. Those in high-rise buildings faced new challenges because elevator riders were restricted to two per car, and the riders could only enter if they were masked and from the same living unit. When individuals needed to be isolated, the remaining members of the household were forced into even less living space and felt additional stress.

Chun and Grinstein-Weiss[50] reported that the impact of housing stress worsened during the pandemic, especially for Black and Hispanic households and among young adults. Specifically, the eviction/foreclosure rate for Black and Hispanic individuals increased by 7 percent, compared with 2 percent for whites. Although African Americans were the least likely group to be forced to move during wave 1 (March to May 2020) of the pandemic, they were almost twice as likely to be forced to move than non-Hispanic white respondents during wave 2 (June to August 2020). Hispanics had the highest vulnerability to eviction in both waves. In terms of age, young adults (eighteen to thirty-nine years) were the most vulnerable to housing-related hardships, followed by middle-aged adults (forty to fifty-four years), then older adults (fifty-five years and older).

The pandemic challenged both individual and collective mental health, but young adults appeared to be disproportionately impacted. For example, Belot et al.[51] studied psychological consequences of the pandemic by age and income in the United States, the United Kingdom, the People's Republic of China, Japan, South Korea, and Italy. The authors measured boredom, loneliness, trouble sleeping, anxiety and stress, and increases in conflicts with family friends and neighbors. The eighteen- to twenty-five-year-old group had the strongest symptoms in all six countries.

As we noted earlier, experience with our college students reinforced the fact that the COVID-19 pandemic literally and figuratively became a nightmare for young people. Government and civic leaders were aware of this problem. In addition to extending vaccination eligibility to twelve- to fifteen-year-old populations, the New Jersey COVID Information Hub[51] was constantly updating information about

- Testing locations, contract tracing, vaccine eligibility, and locations for vaccines.
- Quarantines, limits to indoor gatherings, and travel restrictions.
- Food banks and park access.
- Assistance for people who could not pay their mortgage, rent, utility, and insurance bills.
- Information on what to do in the event of an eviction notice or lost medical care.

The utility of all this information was clear for those who had the ability and means to access it, but it was of less use for many who needed the information the most. County and local governments stepped in to fill the gap. For example, Middlesex County[51] estimated that food insecurity increased from 7.3 percent in the pre-COVID era to 12 percent by the end of 2020. Notably, childhood food insecurity rose from 8.7 percent to 16.7 percent. The county increased its efforts to work with the U.S. Department of Agriculture and food donors, doubling the amount of food it distributed during 2020.

Before COVID-19, New Jersey's poverty rate had been declining.[52] In 2009, the poverty rate was 7.9 percent, rising to 11.4 percent in 2013 in wake of the "great" recession. Then it began to fall back, reaching 9.2 percent in 2019. Boghani[53] reported that the pandemic abruptly ended the decline in poverty. The shutdowns fell heavily on the poor and minorities connected to restaurants, airlines, and personal services. The growth in work opportunities related to port expansions and on-land storage stopped.

New Jersey was not alone in feeling the pinch of unemployment. In April 2020, forty-three U.S. states had their highest unemployment rates since state unemployment data began in 1976.[54] New Jersey lost 757,000 jobs in April 2020, and the state's unemployment rate jumped to 15.3 percent.[55] States with even higher losses were California, Hawaii, Illinois, Indiana, Kentucky, Michigan, Nevada (28 percent, the highest), Ohio, Rhode Island, Vermont, and Washington. Using claims for unemployment insurance for the period of late March through late August 2020, New Jersey reported losses of 10 percent or more for workers in retail, food servicers, entertainment, casinos, gyms, salons, and nonessential health services such as nonessential dental work. These loses fell most heavily on twenty-five- to thirty-four-year-olds without a college degree. Given that New Jersey is more than 90 percent dependent on service-oriented jobs, especially in leisure and hospitality, the pandemic fell like a hammer on the poor and disadvantaged.[56]

The Coronavirus Aid, Relief, and Economic Security (CARES) Act,[57] passed in April 2020, temporarily lowered the poverty rate, especially among children. Married couples received $2,400, and those with children received another $6,500 per child, as well as stimulus checks and relief for the unemployed. Boghani[53] noted, however, that many children remained food insecure.

March 11, 2020, was the day the World Health Organization declared COVID-19 a pandemic. On that date one year later, President Biden signed the American Rescue Plan Act of 2021.[58] The act included direct stimulus payments of $1,400 per person for eligible individuals; included a national strategy for distributing and administering COVID-19 vaccines; extended unemployment benefits; offered grants for small business; provided aid for cities and towns; and included an expansion of the Child Tax Credit to cut child poverty. There was clearly a sense of urgency behind these efforts by elected officials; after some wrangling, it passed a deeply polarized Congress. The trillions of dollars being invested constitute the largest social welfare initiative undertaken by the federal government in decades. Economists predicted that low-income households would benefit the most from the plan—the adult poverty rate could be cut by a quarter, and the child poverty rate cut by half.[59]

Long-Term Health Disparities: Realities and Solutions

Beyond the challenge of returning to some sense of pre-COVID-19 normalcy, the overall follow-up to New Jersey's increased disparity problems are daunting. The state faces some fundamental challenges. One is the reality that climate change is real. Severe weather events not only stress the economy, they impact our most vulnerable, displace populations, and increase disparities. For example, in 1999 Hurricane Floyd battered the state, and at that time it was the most destructive storm in the state's history. In 2011, Floyd's record was superseded by Irene, and then Superstorm Sandy hit, the state's biggest weather-related disaster. Nor will it be the last.

The National Oceanic and Atmospheric Administration[60] has a database of thousands of weather-related events that goes back to 1950. The listed events include wind, snow, rain, thunderstorms, extreme cold, extreme heat, droughts, and funnel clouds. The New Jersey files are not nearly as long as those for California, Florida, and Texas, yet beginning with the year 2000 New Jersey has listed eight tropical cyclones, fourteen severe storms, five winter storms, three floods, and four droughts, each event costing the state at least a billion dollars in damage. For some, a return to their previous living situations after these events will never be possible because they do not have the resources to rebuild nor the ability to remain resilient.

As discussed in more detail in chapter 7, New Jersey, as required, and many local governments in the state have hazard mitigation plans. These plans are supposed to assess vulnerability and propose actions to reduce risk, especially for our most vulnerable. New Jersey has among the best overall state plans for hazard mitigation, but other states (e.g., Oregon, California, and New York) have better plans for handling the cascading events related to an immediate one.[61] Several cities, specifically Portland (Oregon), Los Angeles, and New York City have, we believe, the best local plans. Given the progressive leadership in New Jersey, elected state officials should press for better planning that goes beyond weather-related events. They should consider events like COVID-19 and how such events cascade through the education, housing, and transportation sectors as well as the overall economy (including loss of employment). If broader planning for cascading events fails at the state level, local governments and an active citizenry will need to press for better, integrated plans that address the upstream factors that predict population health. Addressing these upstream factors is best done through a Health in All Policies approach (see chapter 1).

The major solutions to the Spanish Flu pandemic a century ago were social distancing, masks, and handwashing—which should sound familiar. A century later, the tools in our arsenal for the current pandemic include vaccination as well as home screening and early treatments. Government needs to make a sustained commitment to science of all kinds to protect us from preventable events and make us more resilient when events that are not preventable do occur. The annual flu vaccine and pneumococcal vaccination programs have saved many lives, but we still need a national and state commitment to a sustained program of proactive planning and implementation to address COVID-19 and future novel virus outbreaks. Ideally, many science-based projects would originate at the national level and occur in cooperation with other countries. Realistically, expecting international cooperation poses problems, but we need to listen to the expertise of the world's best scientists without being constrained by political litmus tests.

The forces that have led to health disparities existed long before COVID-19 and were exacerbated by the pandemic. Writing for *New Jersey Policy Perspective*, Reynerston[62] argues that COVID-19 proves that New Jersey needs to focus more of its revenue on needy people and small businesses. This, in essence, means finding new tax revenues, placing the state back in a fiscal place with a credit rating that is not further weakened, improving public education funds, increasing affordable housing, building up New Jersey Transit to take on more of a load, and paying into retired worker pension funds. The impact of such actions would require reducing tax breaks for large corporations, easing the reduction of property and estate taxes that benefit more affluent residents, and repealing the 2016 sales tax cut.

In 2020, as the state's tax revenues from income taxes, sales taxes, and corporate business taxes collapsed at an unprecedented pace from the pandemic, the state froze nearly $1 billion in spending.[63] How much will taxes be increased and for how long will large segments of the population tolerate higher taxes and prices? New Jersey may already have passed that point, as documented by the 2020 National Migration Study conducted by United Van Lines.[64,65] New Jersey was the top state in outbound moves for three years in a row. In 2020, 70 percent of moves in the state were outbound. Almost half of those who left the state were high earners ($150,000 or more). New Jersey metropolitan regions also ranked among the nation's top five for outbound moves: Bergen-Passaic (81 percent), Trenton (76 percent), and Newark (72 percent), with those of means noting the COVID-19 pandemic accelerated their decision to leave the state.

What will happen when the call comes to return to yesterday's normal, when national polices again favor the wealthy and state efforts to support the public health sector and address health disparities run out of money? We expect this call soon as the deep, antifederal tradition against big government remains vested. Congress is unlikely to be responsive to calls for sacrifice

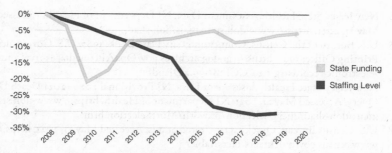

FIGURE 5.1 Cumulative percent change in staffing levels and state funding, New Jersey. Department of Health and Human Services, 2008–2020. (*Source:* Reynertson (2020).[66])

that narrow health and other disparities without a major change in elected officials. What about at the state level? Figure 5.1 shows the state's long-term disinvestment in the public health and human services sectors relative to state funding.

Reynertson[66] reports that, compared with other states, New Jersey was in the bottom quarter of all states for per-person spending on local health departments ($30 per person) in 2019. At the start of the pandemic, the Departments of Health and Human Services were functioning with less funding and about a third less staffing than they had had at the onset of the Great Recession of 2008. While the wealthy and powerful will likely retain sway over the state budget, public pressure must insist on accountability and a Health in All Policies approach in Trenton that addresses public health preparedness and the associated safety net.

References

1   60 Minutes Staff. MLK: a riot is the language of the unheard: *60 Minutes* interview with Mike Wallace (1966). CBS News, August 25, 2013. https://www.cbsnews.com/news/mlk-a-riot-is-the-language-of-the-unheard/

2   Centers for Disease Control and Prevention. General help for CDC WONDER. Updated June 17, 2022. https://wonder.cdc.gov/wonder/help/main.html

3   New Jersey State Health Assessment Data. Mortality and leading causes of death. NJ Department of Health. Updated 2022. Accessed May 21, 2021. https://www-doh.state.nj.us/doh-shad/topic/Mortality.html

4   New Jersey State Health Assessment Data. Behavioral Risk Factor Survey Health Indicator Report Index. NJ Department of Health. Accessed May 21, 2021. https://www-doh.state.nj.us/doh-shad/indicator/CatBRFS.html

5   New Jersey State Health Assessment Data. NJ Department of Health. Accessed
    May 21, 2021. https://www-doh.state.nj.us/doh-shad/
6   U.S. Bureau of the Census. County and City Data Book: 1967. U.S. Government
    Printing Office; 1967. https://catalog.archives.gov/OpaAPI/media/639133/content
    /electronic-records/rg-029/CCDB/199.4DP.pdf
7   New Jersey State Health Assessment Data. NJ Provisional 2020–2021 Death Data
    Query. Accessed May 21, 2021. NJ Department of Health. https://www-doh.state
    .nj.us/doh-shad/query/selection/provdth/MortSelection.html
8   U.S. Census Bureau. QuickFacts: United States. Accessed May 21, 2021. https://
    www.census.gov/quickfacts/facts/table/
9   Raychaudhuri D. The 35 poorest towns in New Jersey, ranked. *NJ.com*, May 15,
    2019. https://www.nj.com/data/2018/01/35_poorest_towns_in_nj.html
10 New Jersey State Police. NJGUNStat. Updated July 2022. Accessed May 21, 2021.
    https://www.nj.gov/oag/njsp/njgunstat/index.shtml
11 Exposing the inequalities of New Jersey's education aid distribution. *New Jersey
    Education Aid* [blog], October 2017. http://njeducationaid.blogspot.com/2017/10/
12 U.S. Environmental Protection Agency. EJScreen EPA's Environmental Justice
    Screening and Mapping Tool (Version 2020). Accessed May 21, 2021. https://
    ejscreen.epa.gov/mapper/index.html
13 U.S. Environmental Protection Agency. Technical Documentation for EJScreen.
    Updated February 18, 2022. Accessed May 21, 2021. https://www.epa.gov/ejscreen
    /technical-documentation-ejscreen
14 New Jersey Department of Health. Top ten cities with highest number of HIV/
    AIDS cases. Updated June 31, 2021. https://www.nj.gov/health/hivstdtb/hiv-aids
    /cities.shtml
15 Centers for Disease Control and Prevention. 500 Cities Project: 2016 to 2019.
    PLACES: Local Data for Better Health, updated December 8, 2020. https://www
    .cdc.gov/places/about/500-cities-2016-2019/index.html
16 Clinton WJ. Federal actions to address environmental justice in minority
    populations and low-income populations. Executive Order 12898, February 11,
    1994. https://www.epa.gov/sites/default/files/2015-02/documents/exec_order
    _12898.pdf
17 Drake J, Charles C, Bourgeois JW, Daniel ES, Kwende M. Exploring the impact
    of the opioid epidemic in Black and Hispanic communities in the United States.
    Drug Sci Policy Law. 2020;6:2050324520940042. doi:10.1177/2050324520940428
18 New Jersey: Opioid-Involved Deaths and Related Harms. National Institute on
    Drug Abuse (NIDA). Updated April 3, 2020. https://web.archive.org/web
    /20210625032058/https://www.drugabuse.gov/drug-topics/opioids/opioid
    -summaries-by-state/new-jersey-opioid-involved-deaths-related-harms
19 Keyes KM, Cerdá M, Brady JE, Havens JR, Galea S. Understanding the rural-
    urban differences in nonmedical prescription opioid use and abuse in the United
    States. *Am J Public Health*. 2014;104(2):e52. doi:10.2105/AJPH.2013.301709
20 Salmond S, Allread V. A population health approach to America's opioid
    epidemic. *Orthop Nurs*. 2019;38(2):95–108. doi:10.1097/NOR.0000000000000521
21 American Medical Association. Issue brief: Reports of increases in opioid-and
    other drug-related overdose and other concerns during COVID pandemic. *JAMA
    Psychiatry*. doi:10.1001/jamapsychiatry.2020.42

22 Substance Abuse and Mental Health Services Administration, Office of Behavioral Health Equity. *The Opioid Crisis and the Black/African American Population: An Urgent Issue*. Publication No. PEP20-05-02-001. Department of Health and Human Services, 2020. https://store.samhsa.gov/product/The-Opioid-Crisis-and-the-Black-African-American-Population-An-Urgent-Issue/PEP20-05-02-001

23 Partners for Women and Justice. The impact of COVID-19 intensifies the shadow pandemic of domestic violence in New Jersey. *ISSUU* [Seton Hall Law School], December 22, 2020. https://issuu.com/seton-hall-law-school/docs/domestic-violence-and-covid-in-nj-december-2020

24 Stolark J. Fact sheet: a brief history of octane in gasoline: from lead to ethanol. Environmental and Energy Study Institute, March 30, 2016. https://www.eesi.org/papers/view/fact-sheet-a-brief-history-of-octane. Accessed May 22, 2021.

25 Centers for Disease Control and Prevention. COVID-19 racial and ethnic disparities. December 10, 2019. https://www.cdc.gov/coronavirus/2019-ncov/community/health-equity/racial-ethnic-disparities/index.html

26 Finch WH, Hernández Finch ME. Poverty and COVID-19: rates of incidence and deaths in the United States during the first 10 weeks of the pandemic. *Front Sociol*. 2020;5:47. doi:10.3389/fsoc.2020.00047

27 Brown C, Ravillion M. Poverty, inequality, and COVID-19 in the US. *VoxEU CEPR Policy Portal*, August 10, 2020. https://voxeu.org/article/poverty-inequality-and-covid-19-us

28 Abedi V, Olulana O, Avula V, et al. Racial, economic, and health inequality and COVID-19 infection in the United States. *J Racial Ethn Health Disparities*. 2021; 8(3):732–742. doi:10.1101/2020.04.26.20079756

29 Kabarriti R, Brodin NP, Maron MI, et al. Association of race and ethnicity with comorbidities and survival among patients with COVID-19 at an urban medical center in New York. *JAMA Netw Open*. 2020;3(9):e2019795. doi:10.1001/jamanetworkopen.2020.19795

30 Seligman B, Ferranna M, Bloom DE. Social determinants of mortality from COVID-19: a simulation study using NHANES. *PLoS Med*. 2021;18(1):e1003490. doi:10.1371/journal.pmed.1003490

31 Bialek S, Bowen V, Chow N, et al. Geographic differences in COVID-19 cases, deaths, and incidence—United States, February 12–April 7, 2020. *MMWR Morb Mortal Wkly Rep*. 2020;69(15):465–471. doi:10.15585/mmwr.mm6915e4

32 Roxby AC, Greninger AL, Hatfield KM, et al. Detection of SARS-CoV-2 among residents and staff members of an independent and assisted living community for older adults—Seattle, Washington, 2020. *MMWR Morb Mortal Wkly Rep*. 2020;69(14):416–418. doi:10.15585/mmwr.mm6914e2

33 Garg S, Kim L, Whitaker M, et al. Hospitalization rates and characteristics of patients hospitalized with laboratory-confirmed coronavirus disease 2019—COVID-NET, 14 states, March 1–30, 2020. *MMWR Morb Mortal Wkly Rep*. 2020; 69(15):458–464. doi:10.15585/mmwr.mm6915e3

34 Doti JL. Examining the impact of socioeconomic variables on COVID-19 death rates at the state level. *J Bioeconomics*. 2021;23(1):15–53. doi:10.1007/s10818-021-09309-9

35 American Association of Family Practice. COVID-19 diagnosis coding explained in a flowchart. *FPM Quick Tips*, July 5, 2020. https://www.aafp.org/journals/fpm/blogs/inpractice/entry/covid_diagnosis_flowcharts.html

36 Orenstein WA. Influenza vaccination: protecting yourself by protecting your community. National Foundation for Infectious Diseases, February 12, 2018. https://www.nfid.org/2018/02/12/influenza-vaccination-protecting-yourself-by-protecting-your-community/

37 Aschwanden C. Five reasons why COVID herd immunity is probably impossible. *Nature*. 2021;591(7851):520–522. doi:10.1038/d41586-021-00728-2

38 U.S. COVID-19 vaccine tracker: see your state's progress. Mayo Clinic. Accessed May 23, 2021. https://www.mayoclinic.org/coronavirus-covid-19/vaccine-tracker

39 Richie H, Ortiz-Ospina E, Beltekian D, et al. Coronavirus (COVID-19) vaccinations by location—statistics and research. *Our World in Data*, accessed May 22, 2021. https://ourworldindata.org/covid-vaccinations

40 NJ hits 1M full vaccinations, with more people eligible. *Associated Press*, March 15, 2021. https://apnews.com/article/health-coronavirus-pandemic-new-jersey-cbfb0 ba68bf86c82970d2fca9d207f5a

41 Conway M, Heller J, Kumar P, Singhal S. A light at the end of the tunnel: US COVID-19 vaccine administration. McKinsey and Company, April 29, 2021. https://www.mckinsey.com/industries/healthcare-systems-and-services/our-insights/a-light-at-the-end-of-the-tunnel-us-covid-19-vaccine-administration

42 Ndugga N, Hill L, Haldar S. Latest data on COVID-19 vaccinations race/ethnicity. KFF, updated July 14. 2022. Accessed May 22, 2021. https://www.kff.org/coronavirus-covid-19/issue-brief/latest-data-on-covid-19-vaccinations-race-ethnicity/

43 Mueller K. These 16 N.J. towns have fewer than 40% of residents vaccinated, Murphy says. *NJ.com*, May 3, 2021. https://www.nj.com/coronavirus/2021/05/these-16-nj-towns-have-fewer-than-40-of-residents-vaccinated-murphy-said.html

44 Stainton L. NJ now shows local vaccination rates. *NJ Spotlight News*, May 11, 2021. https://www.njspotlight.com/2021/05/nj-town-municipal-vaccination-rates-now-online-gov-phil-murphy-says-not-shaming-trying-encourage-meet-july-goal-some-lagging/

45 Vavreck L. $100 as Incentive to get a shot? Experiment suggests it can pay off. *New York Times*, May 4, 2021. https://www.nytimes.com/2021/05/04/upshot/vaccine-incentive-experiment.html

46 Gu Y. Path to normality: 2021 outlook of COVID-19 in the US. Updated April 26, 2021. https://covid19-projections.com/path-to-herd-immunity/

47 Van Lancker W, Parolin Z. COVID-19, school closures, and child poverty: a social crisis in the making. *Lancet Public Health*. 2020;5(5):e243–e244. doi:10.1016/S2468-2667(20)30084-0

48 Hasteltine WA. COVID-19 has exacerbated child poverty, forcing a long overdue policy focus. *Forbes*, March 27, 2021. https://www.forbes.com/sites/williamhaseltine/2021/03/27/covid-19-has-exacerbated-child-poverty-forcing-a-long-overdue-policy-focus/

49 Schwartz AE, Rothbart MW. Let them eat lunch: the impact of universal free meals on student performance. *J Policy Anal Manag*. 2020;39(2):376–410. doi:10.1002/pam.22175

50 Chun Y, Grinstein-Weiss M. Housing inequality gets worse as the COVID-19 pandemic is prolonged. *Brookings*, December 18, 2020. https://www.brookings.edu/blog/up-front/2020/12/18/housing-inequality-gets-worse-as-the-covid-19-pandemic-is-prolonged/

51 Belot M, Choi S, Tripodi E, et al. Unequal consequences of COVID-19 across age and income: representative evidence from six countries. IZA Discussion Paper No. 13366. IZA Institute of Labor Economics, June 2020. https://www.iza.org/publications/dp/13366/unequal-consequences-of-covid-19-across-age-and-income-representative-evidence-from-six-countries

52 Statista Research Department. Poverty rate in New Jersey 2000–2020. *Statista*, November 2021. https://www.statista.com/statistics/205491/poverty-rate-in-new-jersey/

53 Boghani P. How COVID has impacted poverty in America. *PBS Frontline*, December 8, 2020. https://www.pbs.org/wgbh/frontline/article/covid-poverty-america/

54 U.S. Bureau of Labor Statistics. 43 States at historically high unemployment rates in April 2020. *Economics Daily*, May 28, 2020. https://www.bls.gov/opub/ted/2020/43-states-at-historically-high-unemployment-rates-in-april-2020.htm

55 NJ Department of Labor and Workforce Development. Pandemic leads to historic job losses in April [press release]. March 21, 2020. https://www.nj.gov/labor/lwdhome/press/2020/20200521_aprilunemployment.shtml

56 NJ Department of Labor and Workforce Development. Economic brief: New Jersey's changing economy and the recent impact of COVID-19 pandemic. Office of Research and Information, Division of Economic and Demographic Research, September 2020. https://web.archive.org/web/20220403232905/https://nj.gov/labor/lpa/pub/NJ Economic Report 2020.pdf

57 U.S. Department of the Treasury. Policy issues: coronavirus. COVID-19 economic relief. Accessed May 23, 2021. https://home.treasury.gov/policy-issues/coronavirus

58 U.S. Department of the Treasury. Fact sheet: the American Rescue Plan will deliver immediate economic relief to families. March 18, 2021. https://home.treasury.gov/news/featured-stories/fact-sheet-the-american-rescue-plan-will-deliver-immediate-economic-relief-to-families

59 Fowers A, Long H, Schaul K. How big is the Biden stimulus bill? And who gets the most help? *Washington Post*, March 11, 2021. https://www.washingtonpost.com/business/2021/03/10/how-big-is-biden-stimulus/

60 U.S. National Centers for Environmental Information. U.S. Billion-dollar weather and climate disasters, 1980—present. National Oceanic and Atmospheric Administration (NOAA), updated July 21, 2022. doi:10.25921/STKW-7W73

61 Chen J, Greenberg M. Cascading hazards and hazard mitigation plans: Preventing cascading events in the United States. *Risk Hazard Crisis Public Policy.* 2022; 13(1):48–63. doi:10.1002/rhc3.12220

62 Reynerston S. The COVID-19 crisis proves the point: New Jersey needs more revenue to support workers, families, and businesses. *New Jersey Policy Perspective*, March 13, 2020. https://www.njpp.org/publications/report/the-covid-19-crisis-proves-the-point-new-jersey-needs-more-revenue-to-support-workers-families-and-businesses/

63 Treasury freezes nearly a billion dollars in spending as fiscal uncertainty over COVID-19 mounts. Office of the Governor [NJ], March 23, 2020. https://www.nj.gov/governor/news/news/562020/approved/20200323g.shtml

64 NJ tops "most moved from state" ranking again. *New Jersey Business Magazine*, January 4, 2021. https://njbmagazine.com/njb-news-now/nj-tops-most-moved-from-state-ranking-again/

65 Kandell J. Study names New Jersey most moved-out state. *New Jersey Digest Magazine.*, February 1, 2021 https://thedigestonline.com/news/new-jersey-most -moved-out-state/

66 Reynertson S. Years of disinvestment hamper New Jersey's pandemic response. *New Jersey Policy Perspective*, April 20, 2020. https://www.njpp.org/publications /report/years-of-disinvestment-hamper-new-jerseys-pandemic-response/

6

Housing and Education Interventions

———————————————●

> "The past is never dead. It's not even past."
> —William Faulkner[1]

The major theme of Faulkner's novel is spiritual redemption for past wicked deeds through acknowledgment and suffering. Similarly, the New Jersey Supreme Court and plaintiffs in education and housing-related lawsuits made sure that elected officials confronted the suffering of the state's large populations—those trapped in its deteriorating cities while the growing suburbs benefitted from increasing wealth (see also see chapter 3).

This chapter has four objectives:

1   Review the nearly half-century-long history of challenging de facto segregation: the Abbott school district and Mount Laurel decisions.
2   Summarize the New Jersey Supreme Court decisions in the context of the decline of central cities and the expansion of exclusive suburbs.

3 Consider the evidence linking health outcomes to low educational achievement and substandard housing.
4 Review the response of state and local officials as well as the public's perceptions and preferences regarding Abbott and Mount Laurel.

The Path to the Abbott and Mount Laurel Decisions

The 1990s were a pivotal time in the almost half-century-long legal and political struggles to close educational and housing opportunity gaps in New Jersey. The environment that created pressure for legal challenges began in the early twentieth century when immigrants began to settle in the state to work in factories and other supporting jobs. These immigrants were joined by a growing number of migrants who took ferries and newly created bridges and tunnels to commute from New Jersey to New York City and Philadelphia. Along with new highways, federal housing policies, deindustrialization, and other polarizing factors described in chapters 3 and 5, this movement of people led to a marked demographic shift within the state. The middle-class population began moving out of the industrial core areas to populate the state's rapidly growing suburbs.

At the beginning of the 1950s, six urban industrial counties contained the state's largest manufacturing centers in the state: Jersey City, Newark, Trenton, Paterson, Elizabeth, and Camden City. The data in Table 6.1 summarize the changing demographics and distribution of wealth in New Jersey between 1950 and 1980.

Historically, the poorest counties in the United States have not been in New Jersey. In 1979, the county with the lowest income in New Jersey was Cape May, which was ranked 1,510—squarely in the middle of all 3,144 U.S. counties. Yet in 1979 when legal challenges about education and housing were beginning, inequities were already apparent in the geography of family income across the state. Essex and Hudson were among the five poorest counties in New Jersey, along with three in southern New Jersey: Salem, Cumberland, and Cape May. The New Jersey urban industrial core counties were quickly becoming relatively poorer compared with their adjacent suburban neighbors, a key factor behind the impending court cases. The data in Table 6.1 summarize the changing demographics and distribution of wealth in New Jersey between 1950 and 1979.

Table 6.1

State of New Jersey and New Jersey County Comparisons

Area	1950–1960 % Net Migration	1979 % Household Income $ < 10,000	1979 % Household Income $ ≥ 50,000
State of New Jersey	11.9	23.8	6.7
Urban industrial core			
Hudson	−15.2	36.0	2.6
Essex	−8.3	32.6	6.7
Mercer	3.3	24.0	6.4
Passaic	8.1	27.9	4.8
Union	12.4	20.6	8.6
Camden	14.9	26.4	4.7
Adjacent suburbs			
Hunterdon	16.8	3.3	8.8
Somerset	27.6	13.1	10.0
Bergen	28.4	16.6	11.6
Gloucester	29.3	22.1	3.2
Monmouth	32.5	21.8	8.1
Morris	41.7	11.5	12.3
Middlesex	42.3	17.3	6.6
Burlington	45.2	18.1	5.2
Ocean	74.4	28.9	2.6
Outer areas			
Salem	3.3	27.6	2.3
Warren	6.2	22.6	4.0
Cumberland	7.2	31.2	2.7
Sussex	9.1	16.0	5.1
Atlantic	14.2	31.2	4.1
Cape May	25.9	33.9	3.2

SOURCE: U.S. Census Bureau.

As this demographic shift was happening, a wealth belt[2] began to form among the counties in west-central New Jersey, which, along with Bergen County, continued to increase in affluence into the twenty-first century (Table 6.2). The wealth-belt counties quickly replaced the former concentration of wealth in Union, Essex, Passaic, and Hudson counties.

Growing income disparities, along with disparities in educational achievement, housing quality, job opportunities, unemployment, and tax base are what New Jersey's elected officials and the courts saw when they looked closely at plaintiffs' filings. Overall, New Jersey was a wealthy state, but the

Table 6.2

Household Income Ranks of New Jersey
Wealth-Belt Counties, 1979 and 2010

County	Rank in 1979	Rank in 2010
Bergen	46	36
Hunterdon	43	6
Middlesex	66	58
Monmouth	133	32
Morris	14	10
Somerset	16	9
Sussex	93	30

NOTE: Rank 1 corresponds to the wealthiest among all
3,144 U.S. counties.
SOURCE: U.S. Census Bureau.

reality was that it had large pockets of poverty that were separated from areas of increasing wealth by only short automobile trips.

Reducing Disparities in Public Education

The legal challenges related to public school education began with the 1973 *Robinson v. Cahill* case, filed to demonstrate the major differences in school funding. That case led New Jersey to create an unpopular state income tax to supplement local taxes to fund schools.[3,4]

In 1985, the Education Law Center located in Newark filed a legal case against the state of New Jersey's Department of Education, arguing that the public education provided to school children in poor communities was inadequate and unconstitutional per the state's constitution. The "Abbott" in the lawsuit was Raymond Abbott, a resident of Camden who was alphabetically the first to sign onto the lawsuit. Since 1985, more than twenty additional court filings related to the case have been heard by the courts.[3,4] The state Supreme Court's major rulings on school funding have been as follows:

- The education provided to twenty-eight "poorer urban districts" and "special needs districts" was inadequate and unconstitutional, and the state must support a "thorough and efficient" system of free public schools for children five through eighteen years old.

- State resources for underfunded communities were to be equal to those enjoyed by the state's top 10 percent (the wealthiest) school districts to achieve "parity funding."
- Additional state-supported programs would be provided, including paying for high-quality early education, renovating existing schools, and building new ones.

The initial state Supreme Court's principles for selecting an Abbott school district were

- Being among the lowest socioeconomic status districts in the New Jersey Department of Education's District Factor Groups scale (where A = lowest and J = highest status; subject to update).[5]
- Failure to meet the thorough and efficient standard (for example, low performance on the High School Proficiency Assessment exams).
- Evidence of a large proportion of economically disadvantaged students who require more support than provided by a standard public school education.
- Excessive municipal taxes and loss of tax revenues, meaning the local government cannot afford to provide a thorough and efficient education in the school district. Thus, the state must pay.

Using these criteria, the court identified twenty-eight Abbott districts.[6] The court deferred to the New Jersey Department of Education and the state legislature to identify others, raising the number to thirty-one out of the almost 600 school districts in New Jersey.

Since the 1990s, no school district has been removed from the Abbott list, even though several, most notably Hoboken and Jersey City, have gentrified and arguably no longer meet the criteria. Sixteen of the thirty-one are in the original six core counties, including all six of the major manufacturing centers. Seven Abbott school districts are in the most affluent counties, including four in Monmouth (all along the New Jersey shore), two in Middlesex (in former small industrial centers), and Garfield in Bergen County (a relatively poor town in an affluent county). The thirty-one school districts designated as Abbott school districts are found in Figure 6.1.

As early as the 1970s, it was clear that these thirty-one districts were losing people, especially middle-class people. By 1980, only a few years before

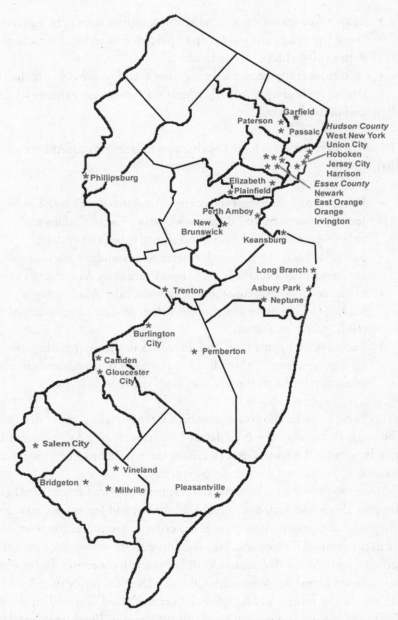

Garfield
Paterson *
*
Passaic
*
Hudson County
West New York
Union City
Hoboken
* * *
* * * *
Jersey City
Harrison
Elizabeth *
Plainfield *
Essex County
Newark
East Orange
Orange
Irvington
Perth Amboy *
New
Brunswick *
* Phillipsburg
Keansburg
*
Long Branch *
Trenton *
Asbury Park *
* Neptune
Burlington
City *
* Pemberton
* Camden
* Gloucester
City
* Salem City
* Vineland
Bridgeton *
* Millville
Pleasantville
*

FIGURE 6.1 Map of New Jersey's Abbott Districts. (*Source:* Education Law Center.[6])

the first Abbott case was filed, about one-third (32.8 percent) of the New Jersey population did not have a high school diploma. In the Abbott districts almost one-half (48.1 percent) had not achieved that status.

The Abbott Programs

New Jersey has invested billions in Abbott programs, particularly for preschool and school construction. Anecdotally, these programs have been called "Robin Hood" education programs in that they take money from the rich and redistribute it to the poor. Some favor this principle as a means of achieving equity in educational opportunity while others do not.

Many people question whether the Abbott preschool program works to increase educational achievement. Barnett et al.[7] evaluated that program, setting the context by asserting that the program has high standards compared with Head Start and other state-funded preschool programs that have a high per-pupil cost. The Abbott preschool program operates on a full school day, has a maximum class size of fifteen, and provides assistant teachers for each classroom. The program hires licensed teachers who are paid on the same scale as public school teachers, and the program offers outreach and interaction with parents.

Additional evaluators[8,9] of the Abbott preschool program have reported an overall half-point increase on a 7-point scale (from fair-good to good-excellent). They expect even larger increases as the teaching and outreach efforts improve. Students show improvements in language, literacy, and math skills. Evaluators also found that these improvements appear to exist at least through the second grade, an expected finding as compared with other preschool programs.[9,10] Another interesting finding is that two years of the Abbott preschool program (beginning at age three) doubled the gains over a single year.

The same group of evaluators followed students through the fifth grade. They reported, "The Abbott Preschool program has produced persistent, meaningful gains in achievement for children in the state's most disadvantaged communities. Achievement gains were particularly large for children who attended the program for two years. Substantive reductions in grade retention and special education placements were produced as well."[10]

As the children moved through grades, however, their relative progress decreased, leading the evaluators to conclude that the Abbott preschool program is not a panacea.[11] They, and others, recommended investments in children before they turn three. Overall, the evaluations showed that the Abbott preschool program's estimated long-term effects are several orders of magnitude greater than less-well-funded and less-organized ones. It was estimated that the program should yield economic benefits far exceeding its costs—measured by building skills, lowering the need to repeat grades, offering special education, reducing crime rates, and other benefits.[12] However, there is no guarantee that the carryover will continue through high school and beyond.

Although a major focus of the Abbott program focused on preschool education, convincing arguments were offered that the physical plant for education in the urban districts was inadequate. The arguments led Governor Whitman to authorize $8.6 billion in bonds to fund the program with an estimated cost of $10 to $20 billion.

Michael Greenberg and colleagues were hired by the New Jersey Construction Alliance to develop an estimate of the economic impact of the construction program on the state's economy (including 251 renovations and additions, and 201 new schools to be built between 2002 to 2015). The estimates depended on the use of union and non-union wages, purchases inside and outside the state, and local arrangements to hire and train workers who live in the Abbott districts. The results estimated that the construction program would generate over $6 billion in personal income, more than $11 billion in gross state product, about $1.3 billion in state and local tax revenues, and about 45,000 jobs.[13]

Chakrabarti and Sutherland[14] reported that the Abbott districts were disproportionately impacted by the economic recession that began in 2007–2008. The researchers compared the Abbott districts with other low-income districts, finding that all low-income districts made cutbacks on support services, but only the Abbott districts cut back on instruction, including laying off nontenured teachers.

In 2008, the New Jersey legislature passed the School Funding Reform Act, which eliminated the Abbott Districts. The state Supreme Court restored aid to the districts in 2011 and blocked the Christie administration's effort to reduce their funds under the New Jersey Schools Development Authority.

In that same year, Governor Christie discussed the state aid for the Abbott districts at a Notre Dame University forum, noting that while the state has 588 school districts, 70 percent of the state aid for education goes to the thirty-one Abbott districts. Weichert[15] reviewed the governor's speech, concluding that it was mostly accurate, indicating that the proportion was closer to 60 percent. For context, the journalist reported that these thirty-one districts represent only 5 percent of all of the state school districts but about 20 percent of the total number of students.

In 2012, Acting Commissioner of New Jersey Department of Education Christopher Cerf acknowledged the remaining gap in educational achievement in New Jersey, despite significant funding in the poorest districts. Noting that in 1973 the thirty-one districts averaged an average per-pupil expenditure of $7,000 (in 2010 dollars), by 2010 it cost $18,850, a cost even higher than in New Jersey's wealthiest school districts.[16] He concluded that the educational gap had not closed and stated, "despite per-pupil spending that has outpaced New Jersey's wealthiest districts and is among the very highest in the country, many of the former Abbott districts remain mired in mediocrity, unable to convert dollars into classroom success" (12).[16] Money, he concluded, "has provided us with moral cover," but what is needed is an educator evaluation system, tenure reform, and other organizational changes.

At the heart of the Abbott cases are clashing values. Should the state be responsible for subsidizing failing school districts? If so, how much responsibility should the state bear? Should state Supreme Court justices be writing policy and managing remedies that normally are reserved for the executive and legislative branches?

A New Jersey Education Aid blog appeared in 2016,[17,18] arguing that the Abbott list was unfair from the start and has become even more unfair. The blog argues that the Abbott list allows a few districts to obtain state benefits and tax relief, whereas equally poor districts get nothing or very little. The blog uses Hoboken and Jersey City as illustrations of two districts that have gentrified and therefore have much larger local resources than they did in the past. The blog also reports that in 1990 former Governor Jim Florio, concerned about the growing inequities between the poor school districts and the affluent ones, proposed the Quality Education Act, which would have reduced aid for affluent districts, required them to pay for teacher pensions, raised taxes overall, and used the savings and tax increases to increase aid for poor and middle-income school districts. Furthermore, the New Jersey Education Aid blog asserts that Florio's proposal was fairer insofar as it did not distinguish between urban, suburban, and rural poor districts and would have elevated the poorest districts funding up to the 60th percentile, not to the 90th.

In June 1990, the blog continues, the state Supreme Court stepped in and removed the opportunity for a legislative solution by rigidly defining the aid process. It concludes that the original Abbott definition was unfair and is now obsolete, notes that several of the Abbott districts, while willing to receive the aid, were offended by the designation and believed that they were delivering a good education.

In addition to the blog, 2016 was the year that the New Jersey Commissioner of Education applied for an order modifying the state Supreme Court's prior decisions in *Abbott v. Burke* (2009) and *Abbott v. Burke* (2011). The application was based on fact that there had been insufficient improvement in student performance, as evidenced by low standardized test results and graduation rates. The court denied the motion, although the decision to deny was without prejudice, which means that the state is not prohibited from raising the same issue in the future.[18]

The Abbott policy battle continues. In March 2019, the Education Law Center[19] reported that twenty-three of the thirty-one Abbott school districts have budgets in fiscal year 2018–2019 that are less than needed to meet the state's "adequacy" level because of shortfalls in property tax revenue and lack of sufficient state aid. The Education Law Center notes that the Abbott districts enroll approximately 20 percent of all public-school students in New Jersey and about 40 percent of New Jersey's low-income students, 54 percent of English as a second language students, and 40 percent of African American and Latino students.

Is there a solution that will be politically acceptable to the Abbott cases that have gone on for almost forty years? Because the courts indicated that sufficient state aid was a "continuing obligation," more legal actions are likely, with the courts monitoring the cases.

Reducing Disparities in Housing

New Jersey has 586 general-purpose governments (counties, cities, towns, townships, villages, and other political jurisdictions), about 1.5 percent of the nation's almost 39,000 general-purpose governments.[20] Yet it is not the absolute number of districts that are important for understanding the Mount Laurel case for reducing disparities in housing. Rather, it is the density of the governing districts that is important. New Jersey has the least amount of land per general-purpose government of any state, which means that someone can drive ten minutes in almost any direction from their New Jersey residence and literally be in a different socioeconomic world.

General-purpose governments are important because they manage local zoning and building codes. The Mount Laurel court cases were filed because many New Jersey local zoning and building codes, whether deliberately or not, excluded poor and middle-income people from finding affordable housing the community. The Mount Laurel case is simply the exemplar of the problem.

Located about a thirty-five-minute drive east of Camden City and Philadelphia, Mount Laurel's population was 2,817 in 1950. The Turnpike was built through Mount Laurel (exit 4), allowing the township's twenty-two-square-mile rural population to increase to 5,249 in 1960, to 11,221 in 1970, and to 17,614 in 1980. By 2000, the community's population exceeded 40,000.

In the 1960s, Mount Laurel set out a plan to change their previously rural community into an upper-middle-income suburb. The zoning for the proposed community included a large, planned unit development and conversion of rural housing into other uses.[21,22] Some of the rural housing units were inhabited by a small Black population, who had roots in the township that extended back to the Revolutionary War. Mount Laurel's plan was to simply remove that population, and they made no plan for resettlement. In fact, the mayor told the small community that if they could not afford the new units, they would simply have to move.[21] The Black community organized, joining forces with the Southern Burlington County NAACP, the Camden County NAACP, and Black and Hispanic residents of the city of Camden to file a class action lawsuit in 1971, claiming local government abuses of power (Figure 6.2). In 1972, the local court agreed with the plaintiffs and ordered Mount Laurel to produce a plan that included affordable housing. The township refused and appealed the decision.[21] In 1975, the state Supreme Court decided the issue in what is called Mount Laurel I. That decision created the Mount Laurel doctrine, which requires local governments to adjust their zoning so that poor and lower-income families have a realistic chance of finding affordable housing in their communities.

The Mount Laurel I decision spurred additional lawsuits. For example, the Fair Share Housing Center (located in Cherry Hill) was formed in October 1975, and it filed cases to demand affordable housing for poor populations.[22] Other cases were filed by the New Jersey Public Advocate and by builders who could build housing that was fully or partly affordable, along with market-rate housing. As the court cases dragged on, they delayed

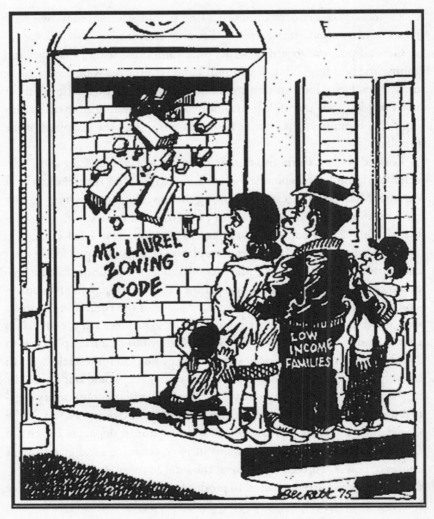

FIGURE 6.2 Cartoon of low-income families awaiting affordable housing under the Mount Laurel decision, 1975. (*Source: What-When-How* (2012).[24])

the construction of affordable housing. In other instances, municipalities changed their zoning ordinances to allow for affordable housing but assigned it to areas unsuitable for residential building, such as near contaminated waste sites, on steep slopes, or within an industrial park.[23,24]

In 1983, attorneys for New Jersey's Public Advocate and others filed a suit addressing widespread noncompliance with the Mount Laurel doctrine. The state Supreme Court issued a decision that every town in New Jersey must provide its "fair share" of the low- and moderate-income housing (Mount Laurel II). The decision also allowed for developers to bring "builder's remedy lawsuits" against municipalities that were not in compliance with its Mount Laurel obligations.[21]

In 1985, the state legislature passed the Fair Share Housing Act, creating the Council on Affordable Housing (COAH). COAH developed a process to determine how much affordable housing was needed and what was to be expected from local governments to meet their fair share obligation. Having the agency assign the number of required affordable housing units was intended to stem the flood of builder's lawsuits that had been filed to pressure local governments to develop a plan for affordable housing. If COAH approved a municipality's plan, the municipality could not be sued for exclusionary zoning.[21] COAH's process also gave local governments credit for rehabilitating existing units and allowed them to pay nearby towns to build half their units as part of a regional cooperative agreement. This option was eliminated in 2008 under Governor Corzine who determined it allowed wealthier communities to opt out, perpetuating segregation and increasing the concentration of poverty in the state's inner cities.

In 1986, COAH provided the rules to build almost 11,000 low- and moderate-income housing units per year through 1993. The second round covered building about 6,500 units annually through 1999. Legal challenges followed, and COAH failed to issue a third set of rules in 1999. The state appellate courts ordered COAH to produce the rules—which it did in 2005, but they satisfied no one and led to more court orders. Paraphrasing a former student who worked with COAH: "We got squeezed from every direction."

On March 10, 2015, the New Jersey Supreme Court divested COAH of its jurisdiction over municipal housing plans. Towns would now petition the lower court for approval of their affordable housing plans. Builders, developers, and other interested parties could intervene in such proceedings, which are known as declaratory judgment actions. One of the most interesting challenges that remained was the accusation that towns deliberately zoned for affordable housing in areas that were environmentally sensitive in order to discourage builders or in areas that would repel rather than attract residents. Author Michael Greenberg was involved in a case where the town claimed it had no open space and instead zoned for affordable housing in a very steep area. He was able to find locations on more suitable land in the same town, which distressed both the town and the developer. We need to point out here that environmental concerns are real, and it is not credible for a town to pick the most sensitive land in their jurisdiction to discourage developers from building affordable housing while finding land for projects that will bring rateables.

The COAH law has had a bigger impact on land use and development than anything since the highway construction boom in the 1950s. People legitimately fear that the historical and cultural heritage of their towns is being lost to outsiders with no stake in the quality of their lives. This cry is similar to those heard from the people who lost their homes and neighborhoods in the Bronx when the Cross Bronx Expressway was built (chapter 3).

Are there solutions to the need for affordable housing? Hills argues that the Mount Laurel decision has not produced the badly needed 100,000 plus houses in the state because, quoting Governor Christie's comment, the COAH criteria are "some arbitrary ridiculous formula that nobody could even explain."[25, 26] The governor's colorful language might be overstated, but the COAH method for assigning a municipality's fair share was difficult to replicate and apply consistently. Hills suggests that a much more workable approach is to have each municipality base their requirement for affordable housing units on typical housing densities. This would allow municipalities to maintain their own land use options so long as they allocate units for the poor and those of modest means. If the municipality could not meet the mandated housing density requirement, it would be required by the courts to explain why it could not.

Marsico[27] labeled the state's approach to providing affordable housing a "40-year failure" and called for the state Supreme Court to manage the process. Behind the rhetoric on both sides of affordable housing issue is the need for the legislature and executive branches to provide a solution that municipalities and poor residents can live with. People with a single income or living on small pensions and Social Security find it difficult to find affordable housing in many New Jersey communities. The failure to find solutions to affordable housing has wasted money on lawsuits, studies, experts, testimony, and arguing about who should make affordable housing decisions rather than facing the quality of life issues inherent in the Mount Laurel cases.[23]

We believe that the Mount Laurel case is different than the Abbott case in one important respect. Nobel Prize winner Daniel Kahneman[28] and colleagues[29] found that people are much more resolute and unyielding about assets that they already possess than those they do not, even if the latter are potentially worth more. Mount Laurel represents local land use assets that people can see. Although Abbott is an expensive statewide program, the wealthier municipalities are not being asked to provide their own land for new schools that will serve outsiders. Thus, we believe the urge to fight against affordable housing requirements has been more highly motivated than the arguments against providing funding for schools in low-income areas.

Health Consequences of Limited Education and Poor Housing

The relationships among health, educational attainment, and housing are anything but simple. Numerous well-written books, reports, and papers have explored these relationships. We begin this section with a discussion of one extremely interesting empirical study that reported a decrease in life expectancy for Americans—a shocking observation for those living in the United States.

Sasson and Hayward[30] reported on the estimated life expectancy for U.S. adults for the years 2010 and 2017. Their population-based study included almost 4.7 million deaths. Recognizing that educational achievement was arguably a major social determinant of health, the authors examined only persons twenty-five to eighty-four years of age because formal education is normally completed by age twenty-five and deaths for persons eighty-five years and older often are multicausal.

The researchers found that the number of years of life lost (dying at an earlier age than expected in the total population) increased among those without a four-year college degree between 2010 and 2017. In other words, people were dying younger in 2017 relative to 2010. By drilling into the data, the researchers reported that life expectancy increased among those who had graduated from college, whether for whites or Blacks, males or females, or other combinations of race and gender. However, white men who had not graduated high school experienced the largest losses in life expectancy whereas Black women with a four-year college degree demonstrated the largest increases. Why did the life expectancy for white men without at least a high school education decline so sharply? The data revealed that drug and alcohol abuse were responsible for almost all of the life expectancy decline.

It is too convenient to assume that more education is a solution to improving health. The cause-effect relationship is not simple. The Virginia Commonwealth's Center (VCU) on Society and Health[31] posits three pathways to explain the relationship:

1   Educational achievement typically leads to higher income, better jobs, social and psychological health, knowledge about health behaviors, and residence in good housing in good neighborhoods. Being healthy increases school attendance, which leads to the ability to concentrate and helps overcome learning disabilities.

2   Poor health undermines educational achievement, often showing up as lack of appropriate eating and physical activity, poor eyesight (inability to afford eyeglasses or even eye examinations), lack of ability to concentrate, low attendance rates, low academic grades and performance on standardized tests, elevated school dropout rates, and behavioral problems.

3   An unstable family environment and stressful neighborhood undermine health and education, especially when instability begins at an early age.

VCU's researchers[31] argue that since the 1980s the association between health and education has intensified. They report that individuals who have not graduated high school are more likely to report being in poor or fair health compared with college graduates (see chapter 2). Between the years 1972 and 2004, self-reporting of poor or fair health among non-Hispanic whites ages forty to sixty-four years old who did not possess a high school diploma compared with those who did increased by 13 percent.

VCU's research group recognized that educational achievement is a commonly used, albeit flawed metric, to compare to health because the data are readily available. However, educational achievement is more than just having a diploma. It typically leads to increased literacy, improved thinking and problem-solving, and healthier behavioral traits. In today's increasingly knowledge-based economy, more education, especially a college diploma, leads to job opportunities. It also leads to higher income and social rank, the ability to buy healthier foods, the time to engage in physical activity, and the resources to pay bills on time, afford transportation, and have ready access to health services.

Bradley and Greene[32] further examined the relationship between health and educational achievement by reviewing 122 articles on the topic. They reported that almost 97 percent of the articles found that health increased with educational achievement. Highly educated individuals are more likely to understand and navigate the healthcare system, allowing them to benefit by taking advantage of what it offers. They are in a better position to detect and treat personal health problems as soon as possible, as well as actively respond to unhealthy conditions and reduce their impact by taking medications and treatment as needed. More education may also improve social engagement skills, help build and expand social networks, and reduce stress due to long-term economic and social hardships. The ability to increase a person's sense of control and to control emotions allows people to reduce their allostatic load— that is, chronic stress leading to increased susceptibility to cardiovascular and gastrointestinal diseases, infections, and diseases such as asthma.[32–40]

Because people with less education tend to earn much less than people with a college education, it follows that poor individuals disproportionately live in more distressed neighborhoods, typically with lower quality schools, poor housing, higher crime, fewer opportunities to purchase healthy food, less open space, and higher levels of environmental hazards. In short, the cumulative evidence strongly supports the existence of a relationship between educational achievement and health status.

The relationship between health and housing may have more accumulated evidence than does any other upstream factor. Yet not everyone is convinced that interventions to improve housing conditions improve health. For example, Thompson et al.[41] went back to 1887 and collected over 13,500 possible studies on health and housing. They selected prospective studies with at least an 80 percent follow up for more than six months, or prospective studies with a control group or other means of controlling for confounding factors. The researchers concluded that the literature is poor, mostly due to small sample sizes and small effects, making it impossible to specify any health gains resulting from housing improvements. We pause here to underscore that the same conclusion can be drawn for the relationship between most upstream factors and health. It is easy to find fault with a study, especially retrospective ones. However, hundreds of studies have concluded that improved housing for poor people will help them become healthier.[42,43]

In 1938, the American Public Health Association (APHA) published its principles of healthy housing. In 2009, the U.S. Surgeon General issued a *Call to Action to Promote Healthy Homes*,[43] followed by empirical assessments of the quantity of inadequate housing. This included 23 million housing units with at least one lead paint hazard, 17 million with indoor allergens, 6.8 million housing units with radon levels above those that require remediation, and 6 million with severe or moderate physical infrastructure problems.[43,44] In 2013, the U.S. Department of Housing and Urban Development (HUD) released its Advancing Healthy Housing: A Strategy for Action that focused on multiple health hazards from allergens and asthma to unintentional injuries and fires.[45,46] In 2014, three-quarters of a century after APHA's original healthy housing book, the National Center for Healthy Housing and APHA provided a new National Healthy Homes Standard.[47]

Notwithstanding the reality that there are relatively few housing studies that are perfectly designed, as a whole Americans spend 80 percent of their time indoors. The disabled, children, seniors, and other vulnerable groups spend even a larger proportion of their time indoors. These facts make it clear that the home environment is a key space for interventions to improve public health.[41,44,48-55]

Taylor[48] summarizes the major pathways that link housing and health as follows:

- Housing quality and safety.
- Neighborhood quality.
- Housing affordability.
- Housing and neighborhood stability.

Quality and safety include conditions inside the residence. Examples of this include lead paint and lead-contaminated drinking water, asbestos, wet conditions with mold, roaches, dirty and pest-infested rugs and furniture, and inadequate ventilation. Inadequate climate control during the coldest and warmest times are risks. Secondhand smoke from tobacco increases respiratory distress, and radon exposure increases the probability of lung cancer. Asthma rates also are widely used as a metric of the relationship between housing and health among children.[56]

The literature appropriately includes neighborhoods as part of the housing–health association. A high-quality neighborhood implies options to acquire nutritious food, a variety of affordable transportation services, and safe places for exercise. The presence of abandoned and dilapidated buildings; unsafe sidewalks and dangerous intersections; parking on streets where bikers, walkers, and scooters proliferate; poor lighting; and a history and threat of crime and segregation are issues. Community groups and local banks and other neighborhood-friendly businesses are sometimes able to help counter some neighborhood problems.

Affordability is a third path linking housing and health. An accepted rule of thumb is that housing should absorb no more than 30 percent of household income. If it absorbs much more, people may buy less food and less nutritious foods, ignore medical warning signals, or not purchase medications. These decisions lead to an increased risk of illness and unhealthy increases in allostatic loads (i.e., the health response due to chronic elevated stress).

Unstable housing conditions are a fourth factor undermining health. Not knowing whether you have a stable residence is a stressor for individuals. As a result, some may become mentally unstable, feel anxious, and turn to substance abuse and violent behavior. Some may be unable to obtain a job because they have no permanent mailing address or access to a reliable answering service. Others may not be able to hold a job, maintain their social network, or receive funds and services from social service agencies.[57]

Public Opinion about Abbott Schools and Mount Laurel

Given the political controversy around these court decisions, we expected to find more polling data than we did. Table 6.3 shows that during the period when the state Supreme Court made monumental decisions in the Abbott and Mount Laurel cases, the public did not have strong feelings about them. When asked in multiple surveys about how the court was doing, about 80 percent of respondents replied "good," "fair," or "don't know."[58,59] Only 20 percent responded "excellent" or "poor." Although the respondents generally lacked familiarity with the cases, the 1987 poll found almost 60 percent supported the Mount Laurel decision.

The Quinnipiac poll[60] of 1,240 New Jersey residents in early 2017 was more informative. Table 6.4 provides poll results for the total group, adding data about self-declared Republicans because their results were notably different from other groups categorized by age, sex, income, educational achievement, and race/ethnicity. The survey results showed that two-thirds of respondents felt that the state Supreme Court was right in ordering the legislature to spend more in poor school districts. A clear plurality favored more spending in poor districts than spending the same per pupil in every district. Two-thirds would support a "millionaire's tax" if the money went to fund public schools. In short, the public supported the principle of providing extra funding to the poorest districts.

In regard to the Mount Laurel mandates, over 70 percent of respondents supported the court's right to require the development of affordable housing, as well as personally favoring more affordable housing. The most interesting response, however, was that 53 percent of respondents perceived that

Table 6.3

Polling Results about the N.J. Supreme Court, Abbott, and Mount Laurel Cases

Question	Date	Option 1 %	Option 2 %	Option 3 %	Option 4 %	Option 5 %
Eagleton Poll						
How would rate the job the N.J. Supreme Court is doing?		Excellent	Good	Only fair	Poor	Don't know
	Oct. 1976 (n = 798)	3	26	38	15	17
	Feb. 1980 (n = 601)	3	25	30	13	29
	Sept. 1982 (n = 503)	3	30	35	9	22
	Sept. 1980 (n = 600)	5	29	30	12	23
	July 1990 (n = 800)	6	31	30	10	24
The Mount Laurel case said that municipalities cannot exclude low and moderate-income housing. Some communities must provide this kind of housing. Have you heard about this court decision?	April–May 1985 (n = 500)	Yes 41	No 57	Don't know 2	NA	NA

Table 6.3
Polling Results about the N.J. Supreme Court, Abbott, and Mount Laurel Cases (*continued*)

Question	Date	Option 1 %	Option 2 %	Option 3 %	Option 4 %	Option 5 %
Do you approve of the Mount Laurel decision?	May–June 1987 (n = 800)	Approve 59	Disapprove 33	Depends 1	Don't know 7	NA
In June 1990, the N.J. Supreme Court decided the *Abbott vs. Burke* case that the state's present system of financing public education is unconstitutional . . . How much have you read or heard about this case?	July 1990 (n = 800)	A lot 16	Some 26	A little 28	Nothing at all 30	Don't know 0
Quinnipiac Poll						
How much have you heard or read about the Mount Laurel decisions?	March 2013 (n = 751)	A great deal 11	Some 14	Just a little 15	Nothing at all 60	NA
Do you approve of the decision?		Approve 52	Disapprove 36	Unsure 11	NA	
How much have you heard about the Council on Affordable Housing?		A great deal 8	Some 20	Just a little 29	Nothing at all 43	

Abbreviation: NA, not applicable.
SOURCES: Eagleton Poll Archive,[58] and Wooley (2009).[59]

Table 6.4
Quinnipiac Poll Results (n = 1,240), February 2017

Question	Option 1 % of Respondents	Option 2 % of Respondents	Option 3 % of Respondents	Option 4 % of Respondents
The New Jersey Supreme Court recently ruled that all New Jersey communities must allow the development of affordable housing for middle class and low-income people. Do you agree or disagree with this New Jersey Supreme Court decision?	Agree Total 71 Republican* 46	Disagree Total 24 Republican* 48		Don't know/ no response Total 5 Republican* 6
How do you feel about having affordable housing for middle class and low income people in your community?	Favorably Total 66 Republican* 41	Unfavorably Total 14 Republican* 31	Neither Total 17 Republican* 25	Don't know/ no response Total 3 Republican* 4
Do you think the community where you live has too much affordable housing for middle class and low income people, not enough, or about the right amount?	Too much Total 7 Republican 14*	Not enough Total 34 Republican* 16	Right amount Total 53 Republican* 64	Don't know/ no response Total 6 Republican* 6
Do you think the state Supreme Court was right to order the state legislature to spend more money to improve the public school in New Jersey's poorest areas or don't you think the state Supreme Court should have done this?	Yes/Right Total 65 Republican* 39	No/Not right Total 30 Republican* 55		Don't know/ no response Total 5 Republican* 6
Do you think the state legislature should spend more tax dollars to improve the public schools in New Jersey's poorest areas or don't you think so?	Yes Total 68 Republican* 44	No Total 29 Republican* 53		Don't know/ no response Total 3 Republican* 3
Do you think the state should provide every school district the same amount of funding per student, or continue to provide more to low-income districts to make up for lower funding through property taxes?	Same Total 36 Republican* 55	Additional funding for poorest districts Total 56 Republican* 36		Don't know/ no response Total 8 Republican* 9

SOURCE: Quinnipiac Poll Release.[60]
*21 percent of total respondents self-identified as Republican.

their communities already had the right amount of affordable housing. Another 34 percent concluded that more affordable housing was needed in their community. Only 7 percent said that they had too much.

In short, the 2017 poll suggests that a clear plurality of New Jersey residents who responded to the poll favored the principles inherent in the Abbott and Mount Laurel decisions.[60,61] Self-declared Republicans were the exception. Two caveats are that this is only one poll and it is our experience that responses about principles change when the economic implications of decisions are explained in detail. In other words, it is possible that the support for these policies is biased by a lack of detailed personalized information.

Summary and Future Challenges

The struggle to build bridges to connect relatively disadvantaged people in New Jersey to growing wealth continues. In 2014, Sharon Lerner reflected on the Abbott cases, including interviewing Raymond Abbott, the first plaintiff.[62] Lerner's conclusion was that Raymond and other Abbott students were fortunate to be exposed to the preschool Abbott programs, and she wonders whether the less well-funded federal No Child Left Behind program of 2001 has a chance of succeeding. In New Jersey, despite the cost and rhetoric on both sides, public opposition to the Abbott program has not been as strong as might be expected. The principle of providing better education for disadvantaged populations seems to be widely accepted by New Jersey taxpayers. Yet the question about whether Abbott works in the long run remains. It is also fair to consider whether the Abbott designation should remain for some districts and whether the relative amount spent on each district is correct. It may take another generation to answer these questions.

The principle of providing affordable housing also seems acceptable for the majority of New Jersey taxpayers. Yet the Mount Laurel cases have produced only a small fraction of the affordable housing that advocates say is needed. Questions remain as to what is fair and reasonable when it comes to providing affordable housing. Do we need to provide affordable units for an ongoing percentage of all persons residing in the state? Or do we need units only for those currently residing in our counties and municipalities? Was the state right to eliminate the option of money transfers between towns to build affordable housing? And, of course, what happens to home rule when the courts—or indeed even the legislature—intervenes?

Developing and implementing policies for public education and afford-able housing are not becoming easier. Several challenges are apparent:

- To date, the burden of addressing education and housing equity has fallen on the state Supreme Court. The composition of the court will eventually change, and its values might shift. Similarly, the legislature and governor could negotiate agreements that could weaken or eliminate the programs. COVID-19, as we would expect, increased the pressure on Mount Laurel and Abbott programs to reduce community desegration.[63]
- Although surveys have shown that the equity principles inherent in the state Supreme Court's rulings are accepted by a majority of New Jersey residents, the principle could yield to repeated political attacks by elected officials. Also, new generations and immigrants may not see the value of the programs to them.
- Ongoing research may show that the Abbott preschool benefits do not carry over after formal education is complete or that projections for affordable housing needs have been overestimated. Conversely, research may show both programs have worked and need to be expanded. Given the more recent attacks on science, some residents may not trust the results of well-designed and well-conducted research.
- Many younger people, empty nesters, frustrated commuters, and new immigrants may choose to live in urban areas, which means the market for affordable housing in the suburbs could shrink. The need would then shift to providing more affordable housing and better schools in urban areas.

The 1950s opened paths to the suburbs and damaged the core cities where wealth had accumulated during the Industrial Revolution. Wealth steadily migrated to the suburbs and the Sunbelt, while northern states such as New Jersey hemorrhaged people and business. Beginning in the 1970s and intensi-fying thereafter, advocacy efforts sought to address the marked education and housing inequities the demographic shift left in its wake. New Jersey made efforts to address these inequities by implementing the Abbott and Mount Laurel policies, which the vast majority of the state's residents consider fair. This brings us to the conclusion that Abbott and Mount Laurel are pieces of the Health in All Policies puzzle. They address upstream factors that improve the overall health of the state, policies that help create a culture of health.

References

1   Faulkner W. *Requiem for a Nun*. New York: Random House; 1951.
2   Hughes JW, Seneca JJ. The emerging wealth belt: New Jersey's new millennium geography. Rutgers Regional Report, Issue Paper No. 17. Edward J. Bloustein School of Planning and Public Policy, September 1999. https://www.issuelab.org /resources/2768/2768.pdf
3   Mooney J. Explainer: *Abbott v. Burke*, changing the rules for funding schools. *NJ Spotlight News*, July 23, 2013. https://www.njspotlightnews.org/2013/07/13 -0710-1649/
4   Goertz M, Edwards M. In search of excellence for all: the courts and New Jersey school finance reform. *J Educ Finance*. 1999;25(1):5–31. doi:10.2307/40704085
5   State of New Jersey, Department of Education. District Factor Groups (DFG) for School Districts. Updated July 15, 2010. https://www.nj.gov/education/finance /rda/dfg.shtml
6   Abbott Districts. Education Law Center. https://edlawcenter.org/litigation /abbott-v-burke/abbott-districts.html
7   Barnett WS, Epstein DJ, Friedman AH, et al. The state of preschool 2008: state preschool yearbook. New Brunswick, NJ: National Institute for Early Childhood Education Research, Rutgers University; 2008. https://nieer.org/wp-content /uploads/2016/10/2008yearbook.pdf
8   Robin K, Frede E, Barnett WS. Is more better? the effects of full-day vs half-day preschool on early school achievement. New Brunswick, NJ: National Institute for Early Education Research, Rutgers University; May 2006. https://nieer.org/wp -content/uploads/2016/08/IsMoreBetter.pdf
9   Frede E, Jung K, Steven Barnett W, Figueras A. The APPLES blossom: Abbott Preschool Program Longitudinal Effects Study (APPLES) preliminary results through 2nd grade: interim report. New Brunswick, NJ: National Institute for Early Education Research, Rutgers University; June 2009. https://nieer.org/wp -content/uploads/2012/04/apples_second_grade_results.pdf
10 Barnett WS, Jung K, Youn M-J, Frede EC. Abbott Preschool Program Longitudinal Effects Study: fifth grade follow-up. New Brunswick, NJ: National Institute for Early Education Research, Rutgers University; March 20, 2013. https://nieer .org/wp-content/uploads/2013/11/APPLES20th20Grade.pdf
11 Bloom HS, Hill CJ, Black AR, Lipsey MW. Performance trajectories and performance gaps as achievement effect-size benchmarks for educational interventions. *J Res Educ Eff*. 2008;1(4):289–328. doi:10.1080/19345740802400072
12 Fitzpatrick MD. Starting school at four: the effect of universal pre-kindergarten on children's academic achievement. *B.E. J Econ Anal Policy*. 2008;8(1):1–40. doi:10.2202/1935-1682.1897
13 Greenberg M, Mantell N, Lahr M, et al. Evaluating the economic effects of a new state-funded school building program: the prevailing wage issue. *Eval Program Plann*. 2005;28(1):33–45. doi:10.1016/J.EVALPROGPLAN.2004.05.002
14 Chakrabarti R, Sutherland S. New Jersey's Abbott Districts: education finances during the Great Recession. *Curr Issues Econ Finance Fed Reserve Bank N Y*. 2013;19(4):1–11. https://www.newyorkfed.org/medialibrary/media/research /current_issues/ci19-4.pdf

15 Weichert B. Chris Christie claims 31 former Abbott districts receive 70 percent of the state aid. *PolitiFact*, December 1, 2011. https://www.politifact.com/factchecks /2011/dec/01/chris-christie/Chris-Christie-claims-31-former-Abbott-districts-r/

16 Cerf CD. *Education Funding Report*. New Jersey Commissioner of Education; February 23, 2012. https://www.nj.gov/education/stateaid/1213/report.pdf

17 The Abbott List has always been unfair. *New Jersey Education Aid* [blog], May 25, 2016. http://njeducationaid.blogspot.com/2016/05/the-abbott-list-has-always -been-unfair_25.html

18 Wilson D. Legally speaking: the return of the Abbott litigation. *School Leader* [New Jersey School Boards Association] 2017;47(5). https://www.njsba.org/news -publications/school-leader/march-april-2017-volume-47-5/legally-speaking -return-abbott-litigation/

19 Krengel S. New Jersey's Abbott Districts: state allows school funding to fall further below constitutional levels. Education Law Center, March 20, 2019. https://edlaw center.org/news/archives/school-funding/new-jersey%E2%80%99s-abbott-districts -state-allows-school-funding-to-fall-further-below-constitutional-levels.html

20 Maciag M. Number of local governments by state. *Governing*, September 14, 2012. https://www.governing.com/archive/number-of-governments-by-state.html

21 Walsh M. What is the Mount Laurel Doctrine? Fair Share Housing Center, November 16, 2009. https://fairsharehousing.org/mount-laurel-doctrine/

22 FareShare Housing Center. About us. https://fairsharehousing.org/about/

23 Kirp DL, Dwyer JP, Rosenthal LA. *Our Town: Race, Housing, and the Soul of Suburbia*. New York: Springer-Verlag; 1995.

24 Massey DS, Albright L, Casciano R, et al. *Climbing Mount Laurel: The Struggle for Affordable Housing and Social Mobility in an American Suburb*. Princeton, NJ: Princeton University Press; 2013.

25 Fleisher L. Gov. Chris Christie proposes eliminating affordable housing quotas, fees. *NJ.com*, May 13, 2010. https://www.nj.com/news/2010/05/gov_chris_christie _proposes_el.html

26 Hills RM. Saving Mount Laurel? *Fordham Urban Law J.* 2016;40(5):1611–1644. https://ir.lawnet.fordham.edu/ulj/vol40/iss5/5

27 Marsico J. A forty-year failure: Why the New Jersey Supreme Court should take control of Mount Laurel enforcement. *Seton Hall Legis J.* 2017;41(1):149–174. https://scholarship.shu.edu/cgi/viewcontent.cgi?article=1113&context=shlj

28 Kahneman D. *Thinking, Fast and Slow*. New York: Farrar, Straus, and Giroux; 2013.

29 Gilovich T, Griffin DW, Kahneman D. *Heuristics and Biases: The Psychology of Intuitive Judgment*. New York: Cambridge University Press; 2002.

30 Sasson I, Hayward MD. Association between educational attainment and causes of death among white and Black US adults, 2010–2017. *JAMA.* 2019;322(8):756. doi:10.1001/jama.2019.11330

31 Center on Society and Health. Why education matters to health: exploring the causes. Virginia Commonwealth University; February 13, 2015. https://societyhealth.vcu.edu /work/the-projects/why-education-matters-to-health-exploring-the-causes.html

32 Bradley BJ, Greene AC. Do health and education agencies in the United States share responsibility for academic achievement and health? A review of 25 years of evidence about the relationship of adolescents' academic achievement and health behaviors. *J Adolesc Health.* 2013;52(5):523–532. doi:10.1016/j.jadohealth.2013.01.008

33   Goldman D, Smith JP. The increasing value of education to health. *Soc Sci Med.*
     2011;72(10):1728–1737. doi:10.1016/j.socscimed.2011.02.047

34   Montez JK, Berkman LF. Trends in the educational gradient of mortality among
     US adults aged 45 to 84 years: bringing regional context into the explanation.
     Am J Public Health. 2014;104(1):e82–e90. doi:10.2105/AJPH.2013.301526

35   Karlamangla AS, Singer BH, Seeman TE. Reduction in allostatic load in older
     adults is associated with lower all-cause mortality risk: MacArthur studies of
     successful aging. *Psychosom Med.* 2006;68(3):500–507. doi:10.1097/01.
     psy.0000221270.93985.82

36   Ver Ploeg M, Breneman V, Farrigan T, et al. Access to Affordable and Nutritious
     Food: Measuring and Understanding Food Deserts and Their Consequences:
     Report to Congress. AP-036. Washington, DC: Economic Research Service,
     U.S. Department of Agriculture; 2009. https://www.ers.usda.gov/publications
     /pub-details/?pubid=42729

37   Brulle RJ, Pellow DN. Environmental justice: human health and environmental
     inequalities. *Annu Rev Public Health.* 2006;27(1):103–124. doi:10.1146/annurev.
     publhealth.27.021405.102124

38   Egerter S, Braveman P, Sadegh-Nobari T, et al. Education and Health. Robert
     Wood Johnson Foundation, April 1, 2011. https://www.rwjf.org/content/dam
     /farm/reports/issue_briefs/2011/rwjf70447

39   Carlson SA, Fulton JE, Lee SM, et al. Physical education and academic achieve-
     ment in elementary school: data from the Early Childhood Longitudinal Study.
     Am J Public Health. 2008;98(4):721–727. doi:10.2105/AJPH.2007.117176

40   National Center for Chronic Disease Prevention and Health Promotion, Division
     of Population Health. Health and Academic Achievement. Washington, DC;
     May 2014. https://stacks.cdc.gov/view/cdc/25627

41   Thomson H, Petticrew M, Morrison D. Health effects of housing improvement:
     systematic review of intervention studies. *BMJ.* 2001;323(7306):187–190.
     doi:10.1136/bmj.323.7306.187

42   Winslow C-EA, Adams FJ, Fouilhoux JA, et al. Basic principles of healthful
     housing: preliminary report, Committee on the Hygiene of Housing. *Am J Public
     Health Nations Health.* 1938;28(3):351–372. https://www.ncbi.nlm.nih.gov/pmc
     /articles/PMC1529239/pdf/amjphnation01005-0119.pdf

43   *The Surgeon General's Call to Action to Promote Healthy Homes.* Rockville, MD:
     Office of the Surgeon General; 2009. https://www.ncbi.nlm.nih.gov/books
     /NBK44192/

44   Raymond J, Wheeler W, Brown M. Inadequate and unhealthy housing, 2007 and
     2009. *MMWR Suppl.* 2011;60(1):21–27. https://www.cdc.gov/mmwr/preview
     /mmwrhtml/su6001a4.htm

45   Ashley P. Advancing Healthy Housing: A Strategy for Action. In: GMA Growth
     and Public Policy Summit. Washington, D.C.; July 17, 2013:24. https://forms
     .consumerbrandsassociation.org/uploadFiles/1B1A9B000002AE.filename.GMA
     _Ashley_7_16_13_pdf.pdf

46   Federal Healthy Homes Work Group. Advancing Healthy Housing: A Strategy
     for Action. Washington, DC: U.S. Department of Housing and Urban Develop-
     ment; 2013. https://www.hud.gov/sites/documents/STRATPLAN_FINAL_11
     _13.PDF

47 National Healthy Housing Standard. National Center for Healthy Housing. Updated September 2022. https://nchh.org/tools-and-data/housing-code-tools/national-healthy-housing-standard/

48 Taylor L. Housing and health: an overview of the literature. *Health Affairs Health Policy Brief*, June 7, 2018. doi:10.1377/hpb20180313.396577

49 Breysse PN, Gant JL. The importance of housing for healthy populations and communities. *J Public Heal Manag Pract*. 2017;23(2):204–206. doi:10.1097/PHH.0000000000000543

50 Pollack C, Egerter S, Sadegh-Nobari T, et al. Where We Live Matters for Our Health: The Links Between Housing and Health. Issue Brief 2. Princeton, NJ: Robert Wood Johnson Foundation Commission to Build a Healthier America; September 2008. https://folio.iupui.edu/bitstream/handle/10244/637/commissionhousing102008.pdf

51 Koh HK, Restuccia R. Housing as health. *JAMA*. 2018;319(1):12. doi:10.1001/jama.2017.20081

52 Kennedy C, Yard E, Dignam T, et al. Blood lead levels among children aged less than 6 Years—Flint, Michigan, 2013–2016. *MMWR Morb Mortal Wkly Rep*. 2016;65(25):650–654. doi:10.15585/mmwr.mm6525e1

53 Fenelon A, Mayne P, Simon AE, et al. Housing assistance programs and adult health in the United States. *Am J Public Health*. 2017;107(4):571–578. doi:10.2105/AJPH.2016.303649

54 Shaw M. Housing and public health. *Annu Rev Public Health*. 2004;25(1):397–418. doi:10.1146/annurev.publhealth.25.101802.123036

55 Adamkiewicz G, Zota AR, Fabian MP, et al. Moving environmental justice indoors: understanding structural influences on residential exposure patterns in low-income communities. *Am J Public Health*. 2011;101(Suppl 1):S238–S245. doi:10.2105/AJPH.2011.300119

56 Schneider D, Freeman N. *Children's Environmental Health: Reducing Risk in a Dangerous World*. Washington, DC: American Public Health Association; 2000.

57 Desmond M. *Evicted: Poverty and Profit in the American City*. New York: Crown; 2016.

58 Center for Public Interest Polling/Eagleton Poll, Poll #65, May–June 1987. Eagleton Poll Archive, Rutgers University. https://eagleton.libraries.rutgers.edu/pollDetail.php?PollNum=065

59 Wooley P. Mt. Laurel, COAH, and the race for governor. Fairleigh Dickinson University, *PublicMind Poll*, March 13, 2009. http://publicmind.fdu.edu/coah/

60 New Jersey voters back court's housing ruling 3–1, Quinnipiac University Poll finds; voters back more state money for poor school districts. *Quinnipiac Poll Release*, February 1, 2017. https://poll.qu.edu/Poll-Release-Legacy?releaseid=2426

61 O'Dea C. Poll finds New Jersey majority favors affordable housing. *NJ Spotlight*, February 2, 2017. https://www.njspotlightnews.org/2017/02/17-02-01-new-poll-finds-nj-majority-for-affordable-housing-but-their-towns-already-have-enough/

62 Lerner S. The Abbott District's fortunate few. *American Prospect*, January 16, 2014. https://prospect.org/education/abbott-district-s-fortunate/

63 O'Connor PK. The Mount Laurel Prescription: The Potential for Public Health Improvement through Community Desegregation in New Jersey. Seton Hall Law, Law Student Repository, 2022. https://scholarship.shu.edu/cgi/viewcontent.cgi?article=2213&context=student_scholarship

7

Acute Natural and Man-Made Hazard Events

————————————————————●

"Risk management is a more realistic term than safety. It implies that hazards are ever-present, that they must be identified, analyzed, evaluated and controlled or rationally accepted."
—Jerome F. Lederer[1]

Humans have survived earthquakes and tsunamis; hurricanes and tornadoes; blizzards, floods, and droughts; plagues and wars; fires, explosions, and train collisions; and other acute hazard events. These low-probability, high-consequence events can lead to loss of life and other harsh consequences for millions of people. This chapter focuses on the challenges hazard events present for the world's mega-urban regions of 10 million or more people. New York and northern New Jersey, along with Tokyo, were the world's first two mega-urban regions. By 2020 there were more than thirty, primarily in Asia. The number could approach fifty by the year 2030. How have social, political, and economic systems and the natural environments of massive interconnected urban settlements coped? This chapter has three objectives:

1 Define acute events, focusing on two issues: uncertainty and cascading effects in dense and interconnected places.
2 Focusing on New Jersey, describe acute weather-related and other natural hazard events; pandemics and epidemics; terrorism and war; and acute events associated with vulnerable engineered and human assets.
3 Review the response of government, private entities, and the public to these threats in a Health in All Policies framework.

Acute Hazard Events

Elisabeth Paté-Cornell[2] (see also Cox[3]) describes "perfect storms" and "black swans" as two images of extremely unlikely but potentially catastrophic events. Perfect storms are aleatory (random) uncertainties. For example, a plume of nuclear material from a damaged nuclear plant will head in the direction of the prevailing wind at the time of the event. That direction may or may not be the usual prevailing wind direction. Because weather forecasting is an imperfect science, the U.S. Nuclear Regulatory Commission requires a fifty-mile wind rose with population estimates for every nuclear power plant in order to evaluate risk because an event may occur at any time. Michael Greenberg and a colleague prepared a wind rose for a proposed nuclear plant to be sited on Newbold Island in the Delaware River.[4] The wind rose showed risk to population centers to the southwest in Philadelphia and to the northeast in New York City. The plant was never built.

In contrast to perfect storms, black swans represent epistemic uncertainty—that is, we lack scientific knowledge about what could go wrong. For example, enormous efforts have been made to understand and control nuclear power plants. Yet the world has learned the hard way that we do not know everything about them there is to know. Paté-Cornell[2] uses the earthquake that triggered the tsunami that led to water topping the protective wall at the Fukushima nuclear power facilities in Japan as an illustration of what we do not know. The wave water knocked out the power supply, and the site then lost its cooling water. The owners and operators did not have enough scientific knowledge to adequately protect the site against the combination of an earthquake and tsunami that produced a fourteen-meter wave. Should they have designed the wall for a higher wave? Should they not have located a nuclear complex in an area with the potential for a major earthquake and tsunami? We learn or should learn from events such as these.

Paté-Cornell[2] also describes the combination of how perfect storms and black swans led to market failures in 2006–2007, resulting in a global recession. She also characterizes the terrorist attacks of September 11, 2001, and the Deepwater Horizon oil platform blowout in 2010, which blanketed the Gulf Coast in crude oil, as low-probability, high-consequence events where randomness and a lack of science contributed to disastrous consequences. Clearly, the COVID-19 pandemic that began in Wuhan in the People's Republic of China was also a low-probability, high-consequence event with a lack of scientific knowledge and randomness.

How much should we spend to manage low-probability, high-consequence hazards? Lederer's thought that opened this chapter is particularly apt: because we cannot guarantee safety, we need to consider risk management as we build more mega-urban settlements that put increased numbers of people at risk. This will be no small feat as Kent[5] believes that the consequences of low-probability events have been substantially underestimated. Ćirković[6] argues that media coverage and cognitive biases lead us to focus on these extreme events only when they are at our doorstep. Thus, planning ahead for hazards like significant earthquakes or large tornadoes may seem like science fiction to residents of New Jersey.[7] This skepticism may be in our residential DNA; consider that on October 30, 1938, Orson Welles's radio broadcast of "War of the Worlds," a story of a Martian invasion in Grovers Mill in West Windsor, New Jersey, terrified some radio listeners who thought it was real. However, Michael Greenberg's father and mother, who had listened to *Mercury Theatre on the Air* every week, found that episode interesting but not frightening—for them, it was science fiction.

Reinhardt et al.[8] developed a probabilistic risk assessment that estimates distribution of serious hazard events over the course a century. They argue that current civil defense measures will help ameliorate some of the consequences of hazard events, but they will not be sufficient. We also note that it is problematic when the powers that be focus only on risk to their immediate constituents and the constituents assume that those in power are working together on larger challenges such as climate change and the risk from meteor strikes.

Consider that the current explanation for the extinction of the dinosaurs is that about 1 million years ago the earth was struck by a large celestial body.[9] The risk of it happening again may be small and random, but it is not negligible. For example, on February 15, 2013, a fifty-eight-foot (eighteen meter) asteroid that weighed about 10,000 metric tons appeared over Russia's southern Ural Mountains traveling at 40,000–42,900 miles per hour. It exploded in the air 18.5 miles above the earth. The energy yield was about thirty times higher than the Hiroshima nuclear weapon in 1945. The asteroid's approach had been undetected, and it caused considerable panic, along with 1,500 injuries and damage to over 7,000 buildings but no deaths.[10]

A single state like New Jersey can plan for some hazard events, but not all. Some events have the potential to devastate large populations and, in the worst case, everyone on earth. These types of events should be joint multinational efforts, which are difficult to organize and manage. After providing a New Jersey–oriented overview of the following acute hazard events, we focus on the first four of these six:

1 Natural disasters, including those intensified by climate change.
2 Uncontrolled infections.
3 Terrorism and war.
4 Infrastructure.
5 Advanced technologies that produce unexpected harm and failed scientific experiments.
6 Invasive species or celestial bodies that strike the earth.

Acute industrial events are included as examples under several of these bullets, and they play a major role in the Cancer Alley presentation in chapter 4.

A New Jersey Perspective on the Worst Acute Events

Michael Warren's 2018 study of the worst disasters in New Jersey since the nineteenth century provides a broad perspective of hazard events.[11] Of his four worst events in the state are two tropical storms and two nor'easters. Hurricane Sandy in 2012 ranks number 1, and the other three are a hurricane in 1944 and nor'easters in 1991 and 1996.

Over eighty events are included in Warren's study, published before the COVID-19 pandemic. The first four categories of events listed here account for 72 percent of his list of worst disasters, and they reflect the state's urban industrial history.

- *Manufacturing and waste management:* Eighteen of the worst disasters (23 percent) were industrial, waste management, or other acute manufacturing events (see chapter 4). The median date for these events was the year 1926. The most recent event was the explosion and fire at Rollins Environmental Services in 1977 in Logan Township in Gloucester County, a facility that managed hazardous chemical wastes. That acute event killed six workers and injured twelve, as well as injuring forty firefighters. The site was rebuilt, and when Greenberg visited the site after it reopened, the adjacent property was selling beautiful flowers that seemed perfectly healthy.
- *Airplane accidents:* Sixteen of the worst disasters (20 percent) involved aviation. The median date for these events was 1951. During World War II, a number of deadly crashes occurred involving military planes. The most recent event on the list was the death of five people in 2011 as they were flying from Teterboro Airport to Atlanta for a vacation; their plane built up ice and crashed on Route 287.
- *Rail accidents:* Thirteen of the worst events (16 percent) were rail accidents involving derailments, bridge collapses, or trains ramming into the back of other trains. In Reed's review of the worst rail accidents in the United States, at the top of the list were two such events in New Jersey in 1853 and 1836.[12] The first involved a collision between two trains running on the same track. The second was a major derailment in Burlington County. Reed points to cheap construction, carelessness, inadequate and primitive communications, lack of brakes in early trains, wooden trains, boiler explosions and fires, bridges left open, wood rails, spring snow melt, and other contributing factors. He summarized early railroading in New Jersey and elsewhere as "many horrors." The median date for railroad hazard events was 1911. Since that time huge investments have taken place in rail transport, yet some rail

problems continue, especially in places where the rails and bridges have not been modernized. The most recent event occurred in Paulsboro Township in 2012 when a freight train derailment spilled vinyl chloride into Mantua Creek.

- *Fires:* Ten of the worst hazard events (13 percent) were fires. The median date for the fire events was 1902, and the most recent was the 1984 Six Flags fire that killed eight of the nine teenagers who entered the Haunted Castle at the wrong time.
- *All others:* Twenty-three of the state's worst hazard events (29 percent) were auto/bus crashes, tornadoes, floods, capsizing ships, construction accidents, and gas main and pipeline failures. Like the others events we have described, very few have occurred in this century.

Warren's valuable study shows that most of the acute events that killed and injured many people in New Jersey occurred almost a century ago.[11] Indeed, the median event date was 1927. Only ten events where more than eighty people were killed or injured have occurred since 1981—that is, over forty years ago. The early urban industrial history of New Jersey is evident in Warren's article, with manufacturing and rail accidents predominating. The two world wars contributed to eight events, including airplane crashes, multiple explosions of munitions plants (including at Picatinny Arsenal in the 1950s, which injured a relative of Dona Schneider), and one terrorism event. We will refer readers to Wikipedia for descriptions of two incidents: the Black Tom explosion of 1916 at what is now Liberty Park and the BOMARC missile accident of 1960 at McGuire Air Force Base. The reader might also recognize "Oh, the humanity!" which was proclaimed by an announcer present when the *Hindenberg,* the world's largest commercial airship, caught fire when it tried to dock at Lakehurst in 1937. These stories are a part of New Jersey's man-made hazard history that we feel need special mention.

Warren's study has additional limitations in that non–New Jersey events that impacted New Jersey residents are not listed. For example, the World Trade Center attack in 2001 killed more of the state's residents than any event listed in Warren's study, but it is not included. Also, the only terrorism incident listed is an explosion of a munitions factory in Kingsland (now Lyndhurst) by German spies in 1917. There are no epidemics or pandemics listed, although human immunodeficiency virus/acquired immunodeficiency syndrome (HIV/AIDS) and COVID-19 have clearly killed thousands of New Jerseyans. There also is no discussion of climate change as exacerbating hazard events, including the costs of property damage and their impact on the quality of life for those in the path of the events. Thus, we must go beyond Warren's historical study to focus on relatively recent and likely future low-probability, high-consequence events in New Jersey and its environs.

Weather and Weather-Related Events

Massive tropical storms and nor'easters have brought water, ice, and snow to New Jersey, leading to severe flooding, deaths, injuries, and property damage. On September 16, 1999, Hurricane Floyd moved north up the Atlantic coast to cause $250 million in damage (in 1999 dollars). The storm track followed the Raritan River into northern New Jersey, causing the area to be a federally declared disaster in nine counties.[13] Readers may recall the massive flooding and fires in Bound Brook, the fire boats rescuing people from their homes, and the failure of the major water treatment plant in Bridgewater, which forced many to boil water for over a week. These events led to the Green Brook Flood Control project at a cost exceeding $100 million. The damage inflicted by Floyd made it the costliest storm in New Jersey history before the twenty-first century.

Hurricane Irene (the "monster storm") hit New Jersey on August 28, 2011.[14] Nine deaths, many injuries, and over a billion dollars (in 2011 dollars) in damages followed. Over ten inches of rain soaked the state, and hundreds of thousands of homes and businesses lost power. Every New Jersey county was part of the presidentially declared disaster area.

Hurricane Sandy hit the New Jersey shore on October 29, 2012,[15] bringing almost a foot of rain and unrelenting powerful winds. The storm killed almost 100 people in New Jersey and nearby areas in New York and Pennsylvania. Over 2 million New Jersey residents lost electricity, many for a week or more, and 300,000 homes were damaged. Some homes could not be saved and had to be demolished. Thousands of residents were evacuated, and some were never able to return to their lost homes. Depression and other psychological symptoms effected many who lost their friends, homes, and neighborhoods.[16] Many of the state's residents wore T-shirts sporting the mantras "Jersey Strong" and "I Survived Hurricane Sandy" to show support for those impacted by the storm and those who came to their aid (Figure 7.1). The estimated cost of Sandy

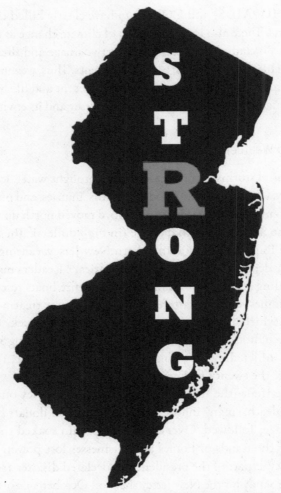

FIGURE 7.1 One of the "Jersey Strong" logos that appeared on Rutgers T-shirts after Hurricane Sandy.

was $30–$50 billion (in 2012 dollars). Since then, more New Jersey homes in flood-prone areas have been purchased under the Blue Acres[17] buyout program, and many shore communities have re-evaluated their land use plans.

Hurricane Ida hit many of the same spots in New Jersey in September 2021, leading to deaths, injuries, and extensive property damage.

Bound Brook, Manville, and other communities, despite major flood control investments, were badly damaged. We cannot say how much worse the damage would have been without earlier flood control investments.

While Floyd, Irene, and Sandy have become household names in New Jersey, we cannot afford to forget the immense effects of nor'easters and droughts. Nor'easters are storms that hit from the northeast, normally bringing heavy rain or snow. In combination with other weather effects, they can be incredibly damaging. For example, Hurricane Sandy was initially expected to head out to sea, but then it collided with a nor'easter that pushed it back toward land where it continued to wreak havoc. Then, one week after Hurricane Sandy had devastated New Jersey, the nor'easter hit on November 7, 2012.[18] Snow fell on a large part of the state causing trees limbs and power lines to become overburdened and break. The combination of the two storms left unprecedented damage.

Michael Baker[19] has reported at least one major nor'easter every year since 2007. New Jersey has not been spared from their damage, including from the Great Blizzard of 1888 that caused 400 deaths in the New York–New Jersey area (nearly all the deaths were in New York). Dove[20] has rated the ten worst nor'easters of all time, and ranked the 1888 storm as number 10. She rated the one that followed shortly after Sandy as the worst, at rank 1.

Droughts are silent but can become acute hazard events. Sponsored by the U.S. Department of Agriculture and the National Oceanic and Atmospheric Administration (NOAA), the National Drought Mitigation Center at the University of Nebraska–Lincoln publishes a weekly virtual map of drought across the United States and subregions.[21] The map presents drought risk according to the federal government's five levels:

- D0—Abnormally Dry
- D1—Moderate Drought
- D2—Severe Drought
- D3—Extreme Drought
- D4—Exceptional Drought

An exceptional drought is a rare emergency. Since 2000, only Salem County and part of Cumberland County have experienced an exceptional drought, during part of 2002. For New Jersey as a whole, the longest drought since 2000 lasted fifty-five weeks, beginning in late October and ending in 2002.[22] The effects of drought are often not immediately recognized, but they are beyond the inconvenience of being unable to wash cars or water lawns. Droughts destroy crops, shrink food supplies, and damage habitats. They increase the risk of wildfires and job loss, reduce options for recreational activities, and increase the risk of heat stroke. For example, in late May 2021, parts of the state were abnormally dry,[23] which meant

- Fire danger was elevated, and the spring fire season started early.
- Crop growth was stunted, and planting was delayed.
- Lawns browned early, and gardens began to wilt.
- Surface water levels declined.

Additionally, the New Jersey Forest Fire Service[24] declared three central New Jersey counties (Burlington, Monmouth, and Ocean) at "very high danger" of fire, with stage 3 campfire restrictions in effect (i.e., all fires prohibited unless in an elevated stove using propane, natural gas, or electricity—no charcoal) and no agricultural burning allowed. The remainder of the state was at "high" danger of fire.

Wildfires are not uncommon in New Jersey, particularly in the Pine Barrens. Hoover[25] writes that about 100,000 wildfires occurred there in the twentieth century, but most did not extend to at least 10,000 acres. The worst wildfire in the state occurred in April 1963, when thirty-seven fires (all originally caused by humans) in the Pine Barrens burned 190,000 acres, killed seven people and destroyed 400 structures. Hoover notes that at least eight significant wildfires have burned more than 1,000 acres in New Jersey since 2000. The worst of these began in Barnegat in 2007, when 17,000 acres of woods in southern Burlington and Ocean counties burned, four homes were destroyed, fifty others were damaged, and more than 1,000 firefighters were called out to fight the blaze.

The chances of more wildfires in New Jersey remain high. For instance, Dona Schneider was driving to get her second COVID-19 shot in March 2021 when she ran into a traffic snarl near Lakewood from a blaze that burned at least 170 acres, destroyed commercial buildings, damaged more than two dozen homes, and left one firefighter critically injured.[26] In May 2021, another wildfire occurred between the Garden State Parkway and Route 9 just northeast of the Bass River that burned 617 acres.[27]

Can the recent acute weather events be attributed to climate change? In 2016 during the Obama administration, the U.S. Environmental Protection Agency[28] published a perspective on the implications of climate change on New Jersey. The federal agency noted that New Jersey has been warming more rapidly than other states: 3 degrees Fahrenheit during the last century. Precipitation also has increased, much of it in the form of heavy rainfall, which makes it difficult to trap for use in replenishing the freshwater supply. Sea level has also risen, and with the ongoing increases in freshwater use, saltwater intrusion into the state's freshwater supplies has increased as well. No one can attribute any single weather event to climate change, although it is tempting.

Hazard events being exacerbated by climate change is unquestionably a serious challenge, especially in densely settled places like New Jersey. Yet many of today's major fires, floods, landslides, and many other "natural" hazards events are anthropogenic in origin or exacerbated by human activity. Two examples include the February 26, 1972, event in Buffalo Creek, West Virginia, that sent a black coal waste slurry down the valley occupied by about 5,000 people living in sixteen small towns.[29] More recently, the 2011 Fukushima-Daiichi nuclear disaster in Japan triggered significant health and ecological consequences, as well as a re-evaluation of Japan's dependence on nuclear energy.[30] There is no denying that both events were a combination of natural and anthropogenic circumstances. Humans designed and built the facilities in locations susceptible to flood and earthquake, respectively, and they were responsible for a less than perfect response to the emergencies.

Enhanced and cascading events from climate change raise the vulnerability of places with dense urban settlement such as New Jersey. In the twentieth century, many people shrugged off hazard events as inevitable—simply a part of the natural cycles of the earth. Now they are characterized as the result of climate change, posing threats to our most vulnerable populations (see chapter 5) as well as representing a war against the next generations.[31,32] Climate shifts also increase threats from some infectious diseases.[33] In 2018, the *Lancet*'s Climate Change Countdown[34] report made it clear that biological agents pose a major threat to the United States and lead to human, ecological, social, economic, and political consequences.

Infectious Diseases

In 2009, New Jersey reported fourteen deaths and approximately 3,000 cases of the H1N1 strain of influenza (swine flu). More than 280,000 persons worldwide died from the infection in that year. In a situation without a vaccine, the recommendations to the public for fighting swine flu were similar to those for COVID-19:[35]

- Avoid close contact (maintain social distancing).
- Stay home when you are sick (isolate).
- Cover your mouth and nose (wear a mask).
- Wash your hands often.
- Avoid touching your eyes, nose, and mouth.
- Get plenty of sleep, be physically active, manage your stress, drink plenty of fluids, eat nutritious foods, and engage in other good health practices.

On April 11, 2020, early in the appearance of COVID-19 in New Jersey, Governor Phil Murphy reported 60,000 New Jersey residents were already confirmed to have COVID-19 infections, of whom 251 died. The epidemiology of the outbreak was also clear. Johnson[36] reported that 78 percent of the early deaths were among those sixty-five years or older, and most occurred among people with pre-existing chronic conditions. That same day, the governor issued an executive order for New Jersey Transit and private companies to cut rail, light rail, and bus service by 50 percent, and to supply their workers with masks and gloves by Monday, April 13.[37] New Jersey schools were closed, as were many other public facilities. Residents were not permitted to gather in groups, and shoppers were asked to wear masks. The effort to reduce the spread through quarantine was unprecedented for many Americans.

A little over a year later, on April 26, 2021, New Jersey reported 875,000 cases confirmed by testing for the virus, and another 123,000 probable cases identified through antigen testing. In other words, almost 1 million positive cases occurred in the state over the course of one year, about one-eighth of New Jersey's population. Also at that time New Jersey had the highest rate of COVID-19 infection of any U.S. state. Chapter 2 summarizes some the likely reasons for the high infection rate of COVID-19 in New Jersey; chapter 5 considers the social and environmental justice associations of the virus; and chapter 8 views the impact of the pandemic as an opportunity to recalibrate health care service in New Jersey.

The Centers for Disease Control and Prevention (CDC) published the major accomplishments of public health over the course of the twentieth century, claiming vaccination and control of infectious diseases as the numbers 1 and 4, respectively.[38] Yet despite the support of the U.S. government in the creation of efficacious vaccines for COVID-19, and the support of state governments in rolling out vaccine programs, we are not sanguine about Congress sustaining funding for these and future efforts. We need ongoing support that will build science that leads to the development of future vaccines. We also need to invest in the surveillance and delivery systems required for public health to prepare for these rare but acute catastrophic infectious events in the future (see chapter 8 for the loss of support for public health relative to the New Jersey state budget).

Terrorism and War

New Jersey has suffered multiple terrorist attacks, although wars have killed far more New Jersey residents. The definition of a terrorist act is found in U.S. Code of Federal Regulations (28 CFR, section 0.85): "unlawful use of force or violence against persons or property with the intent to intimidate or coerce a government, the civilian population, or any segment thereof, in furtherance of political or social objectives." Types of terrorist events include

- Assassination
- Bomb scares
- Cyberattacks
- Hijackings
- Explosive attacks
- Attacks with weapons of mass destruction (biological, chemical, or radiological)

New Jersey and the greater metropolitan region have a history of being targeted for terrorism. New Jersey's 2019 Hazard Mitigation Plan (HMP) lists thirty-one terrorism events in New Jersey and the surrounding area during the period 1905 to 2016.[19] Recent attacks include the February 26, 1993, truck bomb detonated in basement garage of the World Trade Center (WTC), killing six and injuring more than 1,000 persons.[39] The main conspirators (Ramzi Yousef, Ahmad Ajaj, and Mohammad Salameh) lived in Jersey City where they built a 1,300+ pound bomb that exploded in the WTC.

On September 11, 2001, terrorists (part of Osama bin Laden's al-Qaida group) used planes to attack the WTC and the Pentagon, and would have attacked an additional target had the passengers not fought them and caused the plane to crash in Shanksville, Pennsylvania. Almost 3,000 people died in those attacks, and another 10,000 were injured. New Jersey residents accounted for 746 of those who died.[40,41] The longest war in the history of the United States was fought in Afghanistan as a result of the September 11 events.

In October 2011, letters tainted with *Bacillus anthracis* were mailed in Princeton and passed through the Hamilton post office. Five people died and six became sick from the exposures. The assumed perpetrator, microbiologist Bruce Ivins, committed suicide. The Hamilton post office was shut down for more than four years, the facility was scrubbed, and a great deal of equipment was replaced, costing tens of millions of dollars.[42,43]

Additional terrorism events occurred in New Jersey within the last decade. From September 17 to 19, 2016, multiple bombs were planted at the train station in Elizabeth, one of which exploded; a pipe bomb exploded in Seaside Park, New Jersey; and two pressure cooker bombs were planted in the Chelsea neighborhood of Manhattan, one of which exploded. The three exploding bombs injured thirty-one people.[44] On September 19, 2016, Ahmad Kahn Rahimi, a resident of Elizabeth, was identified as the perpetrator. He was arrested in Linden after exchanging gunfire with and wounding a Linden policeman. Rahimi was considered a lone terrorist influenced by the ideology of al-Qaida, and he was given a life sentence without chance for parole.

The state's Office of Homeland Security and Preparedness reports that of the forty-four domestic terrorism incidents in the United States in 2019, four had a nexus to New Jersey.[45] The most egregious of these occurred on December 12, 2019, when a man and woman were stopped by a policeman near a cemetery in Jersey City.[44] They killed the officer and drove to a kosher market where they killed three more people. An all-out gun battle ensued at the market, leaving two officers wounded and the two attackers killed. Later investigations suggested the attack was a hate crime against police and Jews. New Jersey has expanded the definition of a hate crime to include crimes against people based on their religion, national origin, and race.[46]

Lesser examples from 2019 include a Sussex County man obsessed with Nazis and mass shootings who was charged with weapons offenses and bias intimidation, and a Camden County man arrested on accusations that he directed acts of vandalism against two synagogues in Midwestern states. Unfortunately, recruiting efforts for domestic terror groups have more than doubled across the nation since 2018, and the impacts are only just beginning to be felt in New Jersey.[47]

The New Jersey HMP[19] for 2019 includes a section on terrorism. Every state HMP discusses terrorism, but New Jersey's goes into considerable detail for good reasons. The state has valuable physical and symbolic assets to protect. For example, Joint Base McGuire-Dix-Lakehurst, the Meadowlands complex, the Prudential Center in Newark, Atlantic City casinos, the Battleship New Jersey in Camden, and the government complex in Trenton are high-visibility targets. And although New Jersey has lost many of its industrial assets, some obvious potential terrorist targets remain, such as the Oyster Creek and other nuclear power plants, the Kuehne chemical complex in Kearny that produces chlorine, and the state's multiple petroleum refineries and tank farms. Arguably, the Newark and Elizabeth port complex presents the most valuable set of clustered assets in the state. Additionally, New Jersey's transit assets are critical to the national economy, including Newark Liberty International Airport and the main Amtrak northeast corridor line (the longest stretch of Amtrak line between Boston and Washington, DC). Amtrak, along with other heavy and light rail lines, gives New Jersey the largest publicly managed mass transit system of any U.S. state.

Although this section focused on terrorism rather than war, we cannot assume that New Jersey would escape devastation should another war break out on U.S. soil. Nor can we assume that wars of the future will be less destructive than in the past. For those interested in war in New Jersey, there is a history of efforts to land spies and sabotage power plants, the New York City water system, the large Pennsylvania Railroad assets in Newark, and other key engineered systems in the New York City–New Jersey area.[48] Of interest is the fact that Cape May County was converted into a major fortress to prevent Germany from blocking access to Delaware River shipbuilding facilities and petroleum refineries during World War II.[49] Similarly, the Department of Military Affairs and Veterans Affairs[50] lists three war memorials that we encourage citizens to visit as a reminder of the costs of wars that, while not on home soil, have cost the state dearly in human assets:

- The World War II Memorial at Veterans Park (across from the State House in Trenton) reminds us that 560,000 New Jersey residents served in that war and the state was an important center for military training and industrial production for the war effort.

- The Korean War Memorial in Atlantic City honors the 191,000 New Jerseyans who served in that conflict.
- The Vietnam War Memorial in Holmdel honors the more than 1,500 New Jersey residents who died while serving in Southeast Asia.

Vulnerable Infrastructure Assets

All states compete to attract skilled people and maintain an investor-friendly economy. The rail, road, airport, and other infrastructure initially built to accommodate manufacturing, support war efforts, and attract commuters have been New Jersey's most important assets. Yet much of the key infrastructure in the state is a century old or older. It has also been vulnerable to significant degradation. The hazard events we will list predictably found the weak points.

On November 30, 2012, a freight train with eighty-four cars did not make it across a century-old drawbridge connecting Camden and Paulsboro. It derailed, and four cars fell into Mantua Creek in Gloucester.[49] One car containing vinyl chloride (a carcinogenic agent) used to make plastic leaked, and the surrounding area had to be evacuated. This same bridge previously had buckled in 2009 when a coal train passed over it. Even though New Jersey has much less manufacturing than it did a half century ago, it depends on many of the same old rail lines and bridges.

Rail has become an increasingly important asset nationally in recent years because it is the least expensive way to ship bulk cargo over land. An event such as the Paulsboro derailment may be more likely in natural resource–rich areas of the Midwest, South, and West, but it sent a wake-up call to New Jersey to monitor and maintain its older rail and bridge assets. The Paulsboro event was a freight rail example, but we must note that the two weakest rail links in the United States are the Portal (Secaucus) and Dock (Newark) bridges, each a century old—both of which carry massive numbers of Amtrak and New Jersey Transit passengers on a daily basis. Money has been allocated to rebuild these aging structures, but until they are rebuilt, they are potential hazard events with serious human health and economic consequences waiting to happen.[49]

Pipelines are the safest way of transporting gases and liquids.[51,52] In New Jersey some older pipelines without modern technology may be ticking time bombs. As an example, on March 23, 1994, a natural gas pipeline owned by the Texas Eastern Transmission Corporation exploded in Edison, New Jersey.[53] The thirty-six-inch line had been damaged by construction equipment. Fourteen buildings were destroyed or damaged, 1,500 people were evacuated, and one person died from a heart attack. The company did not know that the pipe was damaged, and there was no automatic shutoff valve to control the gas. New Jersey created a "one call" rule, now widely adopted, that requires builders to check for utility lines to before digging. Yet older pipeline sections are subject to corrosion and other failures; nationally, the number of gas and oil pipeline failures has not declined since 2002.

New Jersey has about 1,500 dams, many of which are picturesque and attract tourists. Most were built during a time when it was popular to try to control water for business and recreational purposes. Six dams failed and many others were damaged during Hurricane Irene in 2011.[54] Astudillo[55] reported that more than a third of the state's dams are "high" or "significant" hazards. The dams are located disproportionately in Sussex and Morris Counties, although a failure is not expected to cause the devastation seen in West Virginia, California, and other states with mountains and steep elevations. However, land is scarce in densely settled New Jersey, and new homes are being built downstream from some dams, a land use issue that increases dam-failure-related consequences. Given this vulnerability, the state is working with community groups and not-for-profit organizations to remove legacy vulnerable dams.

Economies expand and shrink—and when they shrink, family and personal violence increase. When economies expand, worker errors, deaths, and injuries increase. During this century, larger and heavier trucks and ships have been introduced to increase productivity. The extent to which these trucks have increased or decreased risk has been arduously debated. The U.S. Department of Transportation almost always concludes that more data are needed. Arguably, larger and heavier trucks and boats do increase risk, but per mile traveled the data vary quite a bit by location, so the risk is not obvious without knowing additional place data.

Transportation failures are almost always due to human error, typically contributed by worker fatigue, improper maintenance, distracted driving, driver inexperience, and improper loading of cargo. Ritchie Law Firm[56] has concluded that 80 percent of truck accidents are caused by driver failures. Hirsch[57] notes that truck-related fatalities reached their highest level in thirty years in 2018, while non-truck-related motor vehicle accidents decreased. Higgs[58] reported that the value of freight moved by trucks in New Jersey is expected to increase 93 percent between 2016 and 2045. TRIP spokesperson Rocky Morley noted that the Port Authority has a massive expansion plan to widen roads and add ramps and special roads to ease bottlenecks.[58] Improving both engineered structures and training is clearly critical if New Jersey is going to increase the value of its massive port asset.

With regard to tankers and cargo ships, a great deal emphasis has been on the safety of double hulls, yet accidents still occur from human error. In the case of supertankers transporting liquefied natural gas, workers must avoid any activity that can cause a spark, avoid oxygen-deficient spaces and corrosive elements, and have long list of other dos and don'ts.[59] Studies show that these expensive, complex vehicles can be too much to handle for stressed workers. The infamous *Exxon Valdez* event in Alaska was attributed to an intoxicated captain.

Human error is also the main explanation for airplane and bus crashes, which can have devastating effects. The media focuses on commercial airplane crashes—for example, the Boeing 737 MAX planes that crashed within five months of each other in 2018–2019.[58] Notably, those crashes appear to have been the product of human failure to train pilots and adequately test computer codes. More generally, however, the commercial aviation industry has become safer. Airplanes and helicopter flights are safer than they were in 1970, technology has improved, and the U.S. National Transportation and Safety Board reports that the majority of aircraft-related fatalities occur in private planes, not commercial ones. Pilot error is the cause in the majority of cases rather than mechanical failure, weather conditions, or other factors.[60,61]

Buses are not as safe as trains, but they are about ten times safer than cars. When buses are dangerous, it is rarely because of the vehicle. Investigations of bus accidents have found that speeding, distracted driving, intoxication, and inadequate maintenance were the major causes. New Jersey has the added vulnerability of high-density traffic with little room to maneuver, and construction projects exacerbate this problem. Other characteristics that increase risk include driver inexperience, weight distribution problems within the bus, and inadequate passenger protection restraints. Despite the higher risk of buses, prices of intercity travel bus travel tend to be inexpensive due to the relatively low gasoline prices that prevailed until early 2022.[62,63]

Solutions in the Health in All Policies Framework

Other chapters have examined polling data to assess public perceptions and preferences for different solutions. This chapter is an exception because acute hazard events are rarely among the public's highest priorities until there is one. Few people welcome hurricanes, nor'easters, terrorist attacks, pandemics, or other events that brutalize populations and destroy their personal and surrounding spaces. Yet consider the difficulty in planning to effectively evacuate large populations, given the roads, settlement patterns, and overall geography of New Jersey. Evacuating our barrier islands in summer hurricane season will become even more challenging in this time of climate change and increasing numbers of extreme weather events. Now consider the impossibility of effectively evacuating the population along a rail line in the most urban part of the state should there be a chemical or radiation leak from a moving train.

How do we plan for these rare events? We elect officials who appoint experts to try to prevent hazard events and help effectively respond when the events occur. Americans spend tens of billions of tax dollars to address natural hazards and some anthropogenic events, but these may manifest in novel forms and at times we do not expect.

The United States is a large and affluent country with a government agency, the Federal Emergency Management Agency (FEMA), and specific line agencies that are responsible for assessing and managing hazards. China recently appointed a Ministry of Emergency Management in charge of acute hazard events, but insufficient time has passed to determine whether this new model is working. Only the Sendai Framework, designed to respond to acute events across the globe and adopted by the United Nations in 2015, is comparable to the U.S. hazard assessment and management model.[64] It is consistent with the idea of Health in All Policies and features a holistic approach to improving health by reducing vulnerability and resilience.

The European Union (EU) put forth its Sendai Framework in 2016.[65] The framework has four priorities:

1 Every EU policy should be risk informed.
2 EU states should use a broad set of policies, from the national scale (e.g., reducing greenhouse gases) to local scales (e.g., building codes), to manage risk, and EU states should involve stakeholders from national to local governance to reduce risk.

3   EU states should emphasize resilience as a priority in risk management investments.
4   EU efforts to rebuild after disaster events should emphasize the
opportunity to reduce societal risk.

The U.S. hazard mitigation process arguably contains many of the same
set of priorities as that of the EU, but they are not as prominent. Like the EU,
the United States has been alarmed by the substantial increase in acute
events with enormous costs. In 1988, with more hazard events occurring,
the United States passed the Robert T. Stafford Relief and Emergency
Assistance Act (PL 100-707), which amended the Disaster Relief Act of
1974. The process tried to reduce the loss of life and property damage by
gathering the best data, using it and information provided by local experts
and outside advisers to assess and prioritize risks and offer plans to reduce
consequences.[66-68] Prior to the Stafford Act, when an event occurred
states would request assistance from the federal government through the
political process. Congress wanted a standardized process to support requests
for federal disaster aid, and it also wanted to reduce the consequences of
acute events. Year 2000 amendments to the Stafford Act required states to
prepare a HMP. Next, grants were provided to local areas to develop plans at
the county, multi-county, and municipal levels. These plans are required to
include the following elements:

- Risk-reduction goals for the area set by scientists, engineers,
  community representatives, officials from public works, police, fire,
  and public health departments, universities, and other sources of
  ideas and data.
- Assessment of the risk of a wide range of hazard events (normally
  semiquantitative).
- Risk management priorities for the area.
- Interorganizational cooperation to set priorities and build support
  for them.
- Meaningful and ongoing public participation.
- Assessment of staff capability to build and carry out the plan.
- Financial needs to implement the plan.

Each local plan is approved by the state government and then by FEMA.
Each plan must be redone every five years. The U.S. process for HMP has

been reviewed, improved, and is considered a work in progress as these plans vary markedly. Several limitations have made most plans a less-than-holistic process that includes all hazards:[69]

- Emphasis on natural hazards and a de-emphasis of anthropogenic ones.
- Neglect of events that can cascade from one hazard event to others (e.g., floods knock out communications and electricity, which undermine efforts by fire and police departments and social services to effectively engage).
- Neglect of cross-referencing with local and regional economic and land use plans.
- Lack of attention to poor, disadvantaged, and special needs populations.
- Unclear processes for accessing the cost effectiveness of risk management expenditures.

Despite these and other limitations, the U.S. hazard mitigation process has been a significant step in establishing a consistent process that considers acute hazard management at the state and local levels.

Another benefit is that the U.S. Department of Homeland Security cooperates with its state and local counterparts. For example, the national government gathers and distributes alerts through social media and more traditional communication mechanisms, which they coordinate with states. The states add their own assets. For example, New Jersey has an Office of Homeland Security Preparedness and a Regional Operations Intelligence Center that operates the state's NJ Alert and Amber Alert systems. New Jersey built a high-tech intelligence center (the Rock) in West Trenton as a central place to manage acute hazard events of all kinds. It is able to withstand strong natural hazards and can shelter staff for an extended period.

Could a framework like Sendai or the Stafford Act make a real contribution during a pandemic such as COVID-19? On September 11, 2020, the UN General Assembly adopted a resolution calling for the application of the Sendai Framework to reduce the risk of the economic, social, and environmental impacts of this disaster. The resolution emphasized the need to invest in disaster risk reduction, to protect and sustainably use ecosystems, and to reduce the likelihood of zoonotic infections and the costs of disasters. UN Secretary-General António Guterres recommended that member states apply the Sendai Framework to ensure a prevention-oriented and risk-informed approach to their COVID-19 response and socioeconomic recovery efforts.[69] Guterres noted that the pandemic had deepened poverty and exclusion while increasing vulnerability and exposure to climate change.

No matter how noble these principles sound, the United Nations has no authority to implement the Sendai principle. In the United States, we will continue to fall back on our federalist principles, relying on FEMA, the CDC, and others to gather information and create and distribute guidance for rescue and recovery to states and communities. Indeed, the COVID-19 pandemic demonstrated the power of state governments to strongly influence the health of their residents.

Summary and Future Challenges

New Jersey has become an affluent, densely settled state with an information- and service-oriented economy. Globalization has nearly eliminated the state's once large industrial base, thereby reducing the likelihood of major acute industrial hazard events but leaving a legacy of sites to be remediated. Investments in rail, road, and electrical power infrastructure have reduced the likelihood of major hazard events. When major events occur, they tend to be triggered by storms and other natural hazards as well as global infectious outbreaks, terrorists, and failed infrastructure. There remain five major challenges to securing the future of New Jersey relative to acute natural and man-made hazards:

1 Without accountability, the HMP process may invest in popular but low-risk projects and ignore more dangerous, plausible acute hazard events.

2 American elected officials and much of the public have exhibited markedly short memories, which can lead to disinvestment in research and projects to reduce the acute risk burden for future generations. Some investments need to be continued, even if no benefits are seen during the next election cycles.

3 A focus on single hazard events ignores the possibility of such events intersecting with others. Vulnerable elements can lead to multihazard events that markedly compound the consequences,

especially in densely settled urban areas like New Jersey. Major cascading events need to be investigated in detail because these have become a reality, not simply frightening ideas spun by science fiction writers.

4   Cooperation among governments and private and not-for-profit organizations is essential to build and maintain preparedness and reduce the potential consequences of acute hazard events. Divisive political postering and positioning threatens cooperation, so it must be set aside for the good of the community of residents.

5   A disproportionate burden of acute hazard events is borne by poor minority populations. To ignore social and environmental justice challenges in planning for future events is disingenuous, at best.

The U.S. HMP process is a good start toward developing a holistic, all-hazards approach for dealing with low-probability acute hazard events. The process has been forged by a history of storms, earthquakes, tornadoes, and other acute natural hazard events where the geography of events is predictable. We need to (1) keep hazardous activities out of vulnerable areas, (2) keep hazards from affecting already developed areas, and (3) strengthen existing developed areas to resist hazards. The path forward for preventing disease outbreaks and terrorism events is less certain, but with strategic investments and planning fewer tragic consequences should materialize. The greater hazard comes of not continuing to monitor and invest in our public health systems because there have been no consequential events for a year or two.

Success requires that the federal, state, and local governments participate in the HMP process, and that every state and some local governments become involved to represent their community priorities. This is especially true for New Jersey where the public health infrastructure is local, representing more than 100 agencies across the twenty-one counties. As we have been told multiple times, home rule can make public health coordination challenging.

Risk assessment and risk management tools are required for planning, but they need not be the most advanced (statistical modeling) ones. The process of HMP has its shortcomings, but it should reduce vulnerability and add resilience elements. We believe that the key is to learn from events, as awful as many of them may be, so we can assess risk and plan for the changes necessary to reduce it. At best, for many places in the United States, reducing acute hazard events will become part of every policy decision (Health in All Policies). At worst, the process will produce plans that are ignored. Our hope is for the former.

References

1 Lavietes S. J. F. Lederer, 101, dies; took risk management to the sky. *New York Times*, February 9, 2004. https://www.nytimes.com/2004/02/09/us/j-f-lederer -101-dies-took-risk-management-to-the-sky.html

2 Paté-Cornell E. On "black swans" and "perfect storms": risk analysis and management when statistics are not enough. *Risk Anal.* 2012;32(11):1823–1833. doi:10.1111/j.1539-6924.2011.01787.x

3 Cox LA. Confronting deep uncertainties in risk analysis. *Risk Anal.* 2012;32(10): 1607–1629. doi:10.1111/j.1539-6924.2012.01792.x

4 Greenberg MR, Krueckeberg D. Population estimates and projections for the Newbold Island region. Newark, NJ: Public Service Electric and Gas Co.; 1972.

5 Kent A. A critical look at risk assessments for global catastrophes. *Risk Anal.* 2004;24(1):157–168. doi:10.1111/j.0272-4332.2004.00419.x

6 Ćirković M. Small theories and large risks—is risk analysis relevant for epistemology? *Risk Anal.* 2012;32(11):1994–2004. doi:10.1111/j.1539-6924.2012.01914.x

7 Greenberg MR. *Explaining Risk Analysis: Protecting Health and the Environment.* New York: Routledge; 2017: chapter 9.

8 Reinhardt JC, Chen X, Liu W, et al. Asteroid risk assessment: a probabilistic approach. *Risk Anal.* 2016;36(2):244–261. doi:10.1111/risa.12453

9 Schwartz MS. What really killed the dinosaurs? Harvard researchers propose new theory. *NPR*, February 16, 2021. https://www.npr.org/2021/02/16/968228310/new -theory-suggests-dinosaur-killing-impact-came-from-edge-of-solar-system

10 Howell E. Chelyabinsk meteor: a wake-up call for Earth. *SPACE.com*, January 9, 2013. https://www.space.com/33623-chelyabinsk-meteor-wake-up-call-for-earth.html

11 Warren MS. The worst disaster in each of New Jersey's 21 counties. *NJ.com*, Oct 20, 2018. https://www.nj.com/entertainment/2018/10/biggest_disaster_in_each_of _njs_21_counties.html

12 Reed RC. *Train Wrecks: A Pictorial History of Accidents on the Main Line.* New York: Bonanza Books; 1968.

13 Giambusso D. Ten years after Hurricane Floyd, NJ towns prepare for future hurricanes. *NJ.com*, April 1, 2009. https://www.nj.com/news/2009/09/ten_years _after_hurricane_floy.html

14 Melisurgo L. Hurricane Irene: recalling a fierce storm 5 years later. *NJ.com*, August 28, 2016. https://www.nj.com/weather/2016/08/hurricane_irene_5_years _later_5_things_to_remember.html

15 Spoto M. Hurricane Sandy continues to haunt N.J. residents 5 years later. *NJ.com*, May 15, 2019. https://www.nj.com/ocean/2017/10/the_fallout_from_hurricane _sandy_5_years_later.html

16 Schwartz RM, Sison C, Kerath SM, et al. The impact of Hurricane Sandy on the mental health of New York area residents. *Am J Disaster Med.* 2015;10(4):339–346. doi:10.5055/ajdm.2015.0216

17 Blue Acres Floodplain Acquisitions. NJ Department of Environmental Protection. Updated September 1, 2022. https://dep.nj.gov/blueacres/

18 Freedman A. Rare November snowstorm strikes in wake of Sandy. *Climate Central*, November 8, 2012. https://www.climatecentral.org/news/snowstorm-strikes-northeast-just-one-week-after-hurricane-sandy-15217

19 Michael Baker International. 2019 New Jersey State Hazard Mitigation Plan. January 25, 2019. http://ready.nj.gov/mitigation/2019-mitigation-plan.shtml

20 Dove L. 10 Worst Nor'easters of all time. *HowStuffWorks*, March 16, 2020. https://science.howstuffworks.com/nature/climate-weather/storms/10-worst-nor-easters.htm

21 Helm R. Drought Monitor (April 2, 2020). National Drought Mitigation Center. University of Nebraska-Lincoln. https://droughtmonitor.unl.edu/

22 Martucci J. South Jersey is officially out of drought. *Press of Atlantic City*, October 29, 2019. https://pressofatlanticcity.com/news/south-jersey-is-officially-out-of-drought/collection_a373982a-aed8-5936-93dd-66dc0e025876.html

23 Melisurgo L. N.J. weather: summer-like heat leaves some areas abnormally dry, sparking high fire threat. *NJ.com*, May 19, 2021. https://www.nj.com/weather/2021/05/njs-summer-like-weather-leaves-some-areas-abnormally-dry-sparking-high-fire-threat.html

24 New Jersey Forest Fire Service. Restrictions Dashboard. NJ Department of Environmental Protection. 2021. https://www.nj.gov/dep/parksandforests/fire/infotools/conditions-restrictions.html

25 Hoover A. 11 Fires that have burned through N.J.'s forests. *NJ.com*, May 15, 2019. https://www.nj.com/burlington/2017/07/nj_forest_fires_through_the_years.html

26 Goldman J. N.J. forest fire that destroyed buildings, damaged homes still burning. Firefighter critically injured. *NJ.com*, March 15, 2021. https://www.nj.com/ocean/2021/03/nj-forest-fire-that-destroyed-buildings-damaged-homes-still-burning-firefighter-critically-injured.html

27 Acevedo N. Rare New Jersey wildfire "was intentionally set," investigators say. *NBC News*, March 20, 2021. https://www.nbcnews.com/news/us-news/rare-new-jersey-wildfire-was-intentionally-set-investigators-say-n1261665

28 U.S. Environmental Protection Agency. What Climate Change Means for New Jersey EPA EPA 430-F-16-032. August 2016. https://archive.org/details/climate-change-nj

29 Erikson KT. *Everything in Its Path: Destruction of Community in the Buffalo Creek Flood*. New York: Simon and Schuster; 1976.

30 Fukushima disaster: what happened at the nuclear plant? *BBC News*, March 10, 2021. https://www.bbc.com/news/world-asia-56252695

31 Connect4Climate. Greta Thunberg full speech at UN Climate Change COP24 Conference. YouTube, December 15, 2018; 03:29. https://www.youtube.com/watch?v=VFkQSGyeCWg

32 Effects of Climate Change on Future Generations. Save the Children. Accessed May 26, 2021. https://www.savethechildren.org/us/what-we-do/emergency-response/climate-change

33 Epstein PR. Emerging diseases and ecosystem instability: new threats to public health. *Am J Public Health*. 1995;85(2):168–172. doi:10.2105/AJPH.85.2.168

34 Watts N, Amann M, Arnell N, et al. The 2019 report of the Lancet Countdown on health and climate change: ensuring that the health of a child born today is not

defined by a changing climate. *Lancet*, November 13, 2019. https://www
.lancetcountdown.org/2019-report

35 Roos R. CDC estimate of global H1N1 pandemic deaths, 284,000. Center for
Infectious Disease Research and Policy, June 27, 2012. https://www.cidrap.umn
.edu/infectious-disease-topics/swine-influenza

36 Johnson B. At least 48% of those who died of coronavirus in N.J. had these
underlying medical conditions. *NJ.com*, April 11, 2020. https://www.nj.com
/coronavirus/2020/04/half-of-those-who-died-of-coronavirus-in-nj-had-these
-underlying-medical-conditions.html

37 Coronavirus New Jersey: COVID-19 death toll rises over 2,000 as positive cases in
Garden State near 60,000. *CBS Philadelphia*, April 11, 2020. https://philadelphia
.cbslocal.com/2020/04/11/coronavirus-new-jersey-covid-19-death-toll-rises-over
-2000-as-positive-cases-in-garden-state-near-60000/

38 Centers for Disease Control and Prevention. Achievements in public health,
1990–1999: control of infectious diseases. *MMWR Morb Mortal Wkly Rep.*
1999;48(29):621–629. https://www.cdc.gov/mmwr/preview/mmwrhtml
/mm4829a1.htm

39 Bureau of Diplomatic Security. 1993 World Trade Center Bombing. U.S.
Department of State, February 21, 2019. https://www.state.gov/1993-world-trade
-center-bombing/

40 Saliba G. Special report: New Jersey—remembering 9/11. *New Jersey Business
Magazine*, September 11, 2017. https://njbmagazine.com/njb-news-now/special
-report-new-jersey-remembering-911/

41 September 11 attacks: facts, background & impact. *History.com*, September 11,
2020. https://www.history.com/topics/21st-century/9-11-attacks

42 Tan CG, Sandhu HS, Crawford DC, et al. Surveillance for anthrax cases
associated with contaminated letters, New Jersey, Delaware, and Pennsylvania,
2001. *Emerg Infect Dis.* 2002;8(10):1073–1077. doi:10.3201/eid0810.020322

43 Duffy E. A decade on, legacy of anthrax attacks lingers in Mercer County and
beyond. *NJ.com*, March 30, 2019. https://www.nj.com/mercer/2011/10/after_a
_decade_the_legacy_of_t.html

44 Larsen E. Ahmad Rahami charged with planting bombs in NJ, NY. *APP.com*,
September 20, 2016. https://www.app.com/story/news/local/emergencies/2016/09
/20/ahmad-khan-rahami-criminal-record/90744590/

45 Rigby P. NJOHSP details New Jersey's threat landscape in 2020 terrorism threat
assessment [press release]. State of New Jersey Office of Homeland Security and
Preparedness, February 21, 2020. https://www.njhomelandsecurity.gov/media
/njohsp-details-new-jerseys-threat-landscape-in-2020-terrorism-threat-assessment

46 Rosenblum AH. Hate crimes in New Jersey. Rosenblum Law, April 12, 2021.
https://rosenblumlaw.com/our-services/criminal-defense/hate-crimes-in-new
-jersey/

47 Maples JM. 2020 Terrorism threat assessment: counterterrorism, domestic,
international. State of New Jersey Office of Homeland Security and Preparedness,
February 2020. https://www.njhomelandsecurity.gov/analysis/2020-terrorism
-threat-assessment

48 Barlow B. The history of submarine warfare off the Jersey coast. PBS WHYY,
October 4, 2018. https://whyy.org/articles/the-history-of-submarine-warfare-off
-the-jersey-coast/

49   DeRosier J. How a German submarine attack forever changed Cape May. *Press of Atlantic City*, July 6, 2017. https://pressofatlanticcity.com/news/local/how-a -german-submarine-attack-forever-changed-cape-may/article_10872806-2fb2 -5907-abee-c07880ac94dd.html

50   NJ Department of Military and Veterans Affairs. Veterans memorials. Updated November 11, 2021. https://www.nj.gov/military/community/civic-engagement /war-memorials/

51   Groeger LV. Pipelines explained: how safe are America's 2.5 million miles of pipelines? *ProPublica*, November 15, 2012. https://www.propublica.org/article /pipelines-explained-how-safe-are-americas-2.5-million-miles-of-pipelines

52   Pipeline and Hazardous Materials Safety Administration. Pipeline Incident 20 Year Trends. U.S. Department of Transportation. Updated June 30, 2022 https://www.phmsa.dot.gov/data-and-statistics/pipeline/pipeline-incident-20 -year-trends

53   Perez-Oena R. Huge Gas Pipeline Explosion Rocks Northeast New Jersey. *New York Times*, March 24, 1994. https://www.nytimes.com/1994/03/24/nyregion /huge-gas-pipeline-explosion-rocks-northeast-new-jersey.html

54   Suro T, New Jersey Water Science Center. Summary of flooding in New Jersey caused by Hurricane Irene, August 27–30, 2011. U.S. Geological Survey, October 20, 2011. https://www.usgs.gov/center-news/summary-flooding-new-jersey -caused-hurricane-irene-august-27-30-2011

55   Astudillo C. 185 N.J. dams could fail in catastrophic flood, but state won't say which ones. *NJ.com*, April 22, 2019. https://www.nj.com/news/2015/10/185_nj _dams_could_fail_in_catastrophic_flood_but_state_wont_say_which_ones .html

56   7 Things you should know about large truck crashes. Ritchie Law Firm PLC, July 24, 2020. https://www.ritchielawfirm.com/7-things-everyone-should-know -about-the-large-truck-crash-epidemic/

57   Hirsch J. Trucking fatalities reach highest level in 30 years. *Trucks.com*, May 27 2019. https://www.trucks.com/2019/10/22/trucking-fatalities-reach-highest-level -30-years/

58   Higgs L. Big rigs are hauling $643B worth of stuff in N.J., and more trucks are coming. *NJ.com*, October 3, 2019. https://www.nj.com/traffic/2019/10/big-rigs-are -hauling-643b-worth-of-stuff-in-nj-and-more-trucks-are-coming.html

59   Frittelli J. Shipping U.S. Crude Oil by Water: Vessel Flag Requirements and Safety Issues. 7-5700, R43653. Washington, DC: Congressional Research Service; 2014. https://sgp.fas.org/crs/misc/R43653.pdf

60   Pappas S. Why private planes are nearly as deadly as cars. *Live Science*, November 7, 2017. https://www.livescience.com/49701-private-planes-safety.html

61   Kreindler Legal Staff. Aviation safety information regarding small private airplane accidents that result in fatalities. Kreindler & Kreindler LLP, March 8, 2018. https://www.kreindler.com/articles/aviation-safety-small-private-airplane -accidents-fatalities

62   Federal Motor Carrier Safety Administration (FMCSA). Large truck and bus crash facts. Updated October 29, 2021. https://www.fmcsa.dot.gov/safety/data -and-statistics/large-truck-and-bus-crash-facts

63   Schwieterman JP, Antolin B, Levin A, et al. The remaking of the motor coach: 2015 year in review of intercity bus service in the United States. Chicago:

Chaddick Institute for Metropolitan Development, DePaul University; 2016. https://las.depaul.edu/centers-and-institutes/chaddick-institute-for-metropolitan -development/research-and-publications/Documents/2015%20Year%20in%20 Review%20of%20Intercity%20Bus%20Service%20in%20the%20United%20 States-110116.pdf

64 Sendai Framework for Disaster Risk Reduction 2015–2030. United Nations Office for Disaster Risk Reduction (UNDRR); 2015. https://www.preventionweb.net /files/43291_sendaiframeworkfordrren.pdf

65 European Civil Protection and Humanitarian Aid Operations. Disaster prepared- ness: factsheet. European Union (EU), 2021. https://ec.europa.eu/echo/what /humanitarian-aid/disaster_preparedness_en

66 Schwab J. Hazard Mitigation: Integrating Best Practices into Planning. American Planning Association, Planning Advisory Service, May 1, 2010. https://www .planning.org/publications/report/9026884/

67 American Planning Association. Hazards Planning Center: Planning Information Exchange. Updated July 25, 2022. https://www.planning.org/nationalcenters/hazards /planninginformationexchange/

68 Federal Emergency Management Agency. Hazard Mitigation Planning. Depart- ment of Homeland Security, FEMA. Updated August 18, 2022. https://www.fema .gov/emergency-managers/risk-management/hazard-mitigation-planning

69 Chen J, Greenberg M. Cascading hazards and hazard mitigation plans: preventing cascading events in the United States. *Risk Hazards Crisis Public Pol.* 2022;13(1): 48–63. doi:10.1002/rhc3.12220

8

Reshuffling Health Care

————————————————————●

> "America's healthcare system is neither
> healthy, caring, nor a system."
> —Walter Cronkite[1]

Walter Cronkite's mid-twentieth century observation remains relevant today. Despite the addition of Medicare, Medicaid, the Affordable Care Act of 2010 (ACA, popularly called Obamacare) and the Children's Health Insurance Program (CHIP), the nation still does not have a system of accessible health care that covers everyone. Instead, the public is served by a patchwork of public and private insurance programs that are confusing, with co-pays and restrictions that are ever changing. Despite the fact that a universal system is not yet on the horizon, there is a slow but sure shift happening in health care. Both public and private insurance programs now recognize that investing in prevention is more profitable than paying for treatments.

This chapter has four objectives:

1 Review the history of health care access in the United States since the mid-1950s.
2 Evaluate evidence linking healthcare access with health outcomes.

3 Describe recent attempts to lower direct healthcare costs.
4 Consider how upstream responses to improving population health can lower healthcare costs, with an eye to the future.

The Healthcare Timeline

American healthcare policy is widely acknowledged as beginning with the Hill-Burton Act of 1946. The Act gave hospitals, nursing homes and other healthcare facilities grants for both new construction and modernization. Rural communities were also guaranteed access to hospital care when the Surgeon General established a hospital bed to patient ratio of 4.5 beds per 1,000 population.[2] In return for Hill-Burton funding, facilities agreed to provide health care for all individuals in their community regardless of the ability to pay. This requirement was shortsighted because it did not address how facilities funded by Hill-Burton could continue to provide mandated services to those who could not pay after the federal funding ceased.[3]

As of 2020, 131 facilities have remained on the list of Hill-Burton obligated facilities. Five of them are located in New Jersey: one is a general hospital (Jersey City Medical Center), two are outpatient facilities (Metropolitan Family Health Center in Jersey City and Paterson Community Health Center), and two are nursing homes in Newark (Broadway House Continuing Care and Spectrum AIDS Day Care).[4] Free care continues to be provided to those who apply and have an income at or below the federal poverty guidelines. Reduced-cost care is provided if an individual's income is up to two times the guidelines (three times for nursing home care).

Hill-Burton is not the only legislation protecting those who require medical care but have no means to pay for it. New Jersey statute 26:2H-18.64 states, "No hospital shall deny any admission or appropriate service to a patient on the basis of that patient's ability to pay or source of payment." There is a $10,000 penalty for each violation.[5] To help pay for this unfunded mandate, New Jersey passed the Charity Care Law in 1978, which allows hospitals to add an "allowable financial element" to help cover uncompensated care and bad debt. The surcharges were increased in accordance with how much uncompensated care a hospital provided, which motivated those with insurance to seek hospitals with less uncompensated care. To address this disparity, the state created the Uncompensated Care Trust Fund, but the solution was imperfect because healthcare costs continued to rise.[6] Today, charity care is covered by the NJ Hospital Care Payment Assistance Program and reimbursed based on the Medicaid payment rate.[7]

In 1986, Congress passed the Emergency Medical Treatment and Active Labor Act (EMTALA) for all hospitals that participate in Medicare (98 percent of all hospitals).[8] EMTALA requires all hospitals with emergency facilities to screen and stabilize patients experiencing emergency conditions before transferring them to another hospital or facility. Hospitals with specialized capabilities, such as a burn unit or neonatal intensive care, are required to accept transfers of patients requiring such services even if that hospital has no emergency department. EMTALA was designed to prevent the "dumping" of indigent patients onto public or charity hospitals, and it also serves as an unfunded mandate that increases hospital costs for emergency services. Some EMTALA patients may require inpatient admission followed by lengthy, costly care which will not be compensated. New Jersey has additional regulations describing the circumstances of how such transfers can be made and by whom.[9]

Rising Costs

The cost of hospital care rose dramatically after Hill-Burton, and by the 1960s the number of insurance companies grew to more than 700. The number of doctors claiming to be full-time specialists increased, leaving a perceived doctor shortage for primary care.[10] With insurance linked to employment and with skyrocketing costs, the uninsured, the poor, and the elderly could no longer afford the levels of health care they needed. Efforts to provide health insurance for at least one of those populations, those aged sixty-five and older, began with the Truman administration but failed in Congress. A second attempt was made by the Kennedy administration, and that, too, failed. Each time, the American Medical Association (AMA) spent millions to block the bills, characterizing the legislation as "socialized medicine" and un-American. These challenges were finally overcome in 1965 when President Lyndon Johnson added the importance of addressing health care in his State of the Union address. A few weeks later, Johnson pressed Congress hard to pass Medicare and Medicaid. He signed the bills into law at the Harry S. Truman Library in Independence, Missouri. In attendance were President Truman and his wife, Bess. Upon signing, Johnson presented eighty-one-year-old Truman and Bess with Medicare cards, numbers 1 and 2.[11,12]

The creation of Medicare and Medicaid helped increase the demand for health care during the 1960s, and the costs the legislation generated were greater than expected. An aging population with Medicare insurance, along with an increase in the number of specialty physicians and in hospital costs, drove American health care to a crisis of unrealistic expectations.[10] Physicians were trained to cure, or at least prevent death, and the loss of a patient, even one of advanced age, was perceived as a personal failure. Patients and their loved ones came to expect the most intensive treatments, even if the patient had no hope of recovery and was kept alive only with the use of a ventilator.[9]

Both physicians and patients believed that more care was better care, so the problem became how to curb unrealistic expectations, particularly at the end of life. Some argued that the answer was to limit the number of physicians. Kenneth Arrow's foundational work in this area cautioned that attempting to ration care by limiting the number of medical school admissions or restricting the number of physician licenses would not be effective in controlling costs. Instead, it would likely increase the incomes of currently practicing physicians.[13]

Also, at the same time it was obvious that the pool of physicians was overwhelmingly male. Medical schools responded by changing their admissions practices. At the beginning of the 1970s, women were 9 percent of medical school admissions. By the end of that decade, they were 25 percent. In 2019, women accounted for 50.5 percent of all medical school students.[14] It was assumed that women would be more inclined to primary practice than would men, and with fewer specialists the physician costs would go down. There was also the unspoken assumption that women physicians would draw lower salaries than men. This has turned out to be true: women practicing primary care in 2020 still earned, on average, 25 percent less than their male colleagues in the same field.[15]

Beginning in 1965, federal funding for medical residencies became available as part of the Social Security Act. Congress ignored Arrow's warning and, as part of the Balanced Budget Act of 1997, capped the number and geographic distribution of Medicare-funded residencies among existing graduate medical education programs at 1996 levels.[9] The cap created a serious problem for staffing hospitals: the number of residency slots was no longer sufficient to permit newly trained physicians to enter the workforce, to replace those who were approaching retirement, to compensate for population shifts, or to cover services for rural and underserved communities.

The Association of American Medical Colleges predicted that New Jersey could be short up to 2,800 physicians by 2022 due to its growing aging population. In response, Congress raised the cap that limits residencies for new physicians on December 23, 2020, a time when the COVID-19 pandemic had stretched hospital resources beyond their capacity. The legislation provides 1,000 new Medicare-supported residency positions, particularly for teaching hospitals in rural areas, in states with new medical schools (New Jersey opened Hackensack Meridian School of Medicine at Seton Hall University in 2018) and hospitals that care for underserved communities.[16]

If controlling the number of physicians was not the solution for controlling increasing healthcare costs, perhaps the fee-for-service model was. Insurance companies complained that physicians were exploiting the system and sought to negotiate "capitation" contracts where they would provide a flat fee for each patient covered rather than reimbursing for individual services. Hospitals also complained that the administrative costs of insurers were excessive and that this was a driver of increased healthcare costs. The hospitals were not wrong. A study in 2017 showed that costs for administering Medicare were 1.4 percent, and those for private insurers averaged 12.3 percent.[17] In an effort to shift the payment system away from fee-for-service, President Nixon signed the Health Maintenance Organization Act of 1973. There were hopes that this model would help bring healthcare costs under control; however, the greater use of technology and medications along with increased hospital and administrative costs and an aging population overwhelmed the effort.

In 1980, New Jersey shifted its healthcare reimbursement system from one based on treatment to one based on diagnosis (Diagnostic Related Group or DRG). The state set DRG rates, and hospitals were encouraged to improve efficiency so that they could retain the difference between their costs and fixed DRG reimbursements. Hospitals were also encouraged to monitor and redirect physician behavior as well as other resource use in order to lower treatment costs. The New Jersey experiment with DRGs became the basis for national policy when the Reagan administration shifted Medicare reimbursements to a DRG system in 1983.[18] Private insurance plans quickly followed.

By 1991, the issue of uncompensated care (charity care plus bad debt) as well as the proliferation of high-technology medical equipment such as magnetic resonance imaging machines made it clear that ongoing reform was needed to curb rising healthcare costs. New Jersey's Health Care Cost Reduction Act of 1991 placed a limit on the surcharges that hospitals could place on their bills and tightened the Certificate of Need (CON) process. In 1992, Judge Wolin (Federal District Court, Newark) upheld a ruling that the federal Employee Retirement Income Security Act (ERISA) precluded some provisions of the DRG system. Specifically, there could no longer be surcharges on insurance bills to cover charity care, hospital bad debt, and Medicare funding shortfalls.[19] Trenton reacted to the Wolin ruling quickly, and the bipartisan Health Care Reform Act of 1992 resulted in several changes. It terminated state rate setting and put the onus on hospitals to negotiate their own DRGs with insurers. Health benefits packages were required to cover necessary and appropriate services, including prevention and primary care. Insurance premiums for small groups were to reflect the larger community rating, and a subsidized insurance program fund was established to aid those without insurance. It also removed the CON process.[19]

Removal of the requirement for a CON to open new facilities led to the proliferation of ambulatory surgery centers and facilities focused on high-tech diagnostic and treatment services. Both hospitals and medical groups found they could make more money on outpatient services than treating inpatients. To control costs and take advantage of the new payment system, hospitals took the additional step of beginning to consolidate—the start of the corporatization of health care.[10]

Additional federal legislation aimed at creating or securing access to health care and medications through insurance vehicles was passed in the following Clinton, George W. Bush, and Obama administrations (Table 8.1), but a unifying system of health care that would cover all citizens was not achieved. At the time of this writing, the concept of "Medicare for All" appears to be in limbo.

Linking Health Care with Health Outcomes

It may surprise some to learn that utilization of healthcare services does not necessarily equate with good health outcomes. In 1973, Wennberg and Gittelsohn wrote a classic article on this topic.[20] They found that patients with similar illnesses received different types and amounts of health care based on their geographic location in the various hospital service areas of Vermont. More than two decades of follow-up data showed that spending more on

Table 8.1

Timeline of Health Care Legislation in the United States

Date	Legislation	Impact
1965	President Johnson signed Titles XVIII (Medicare) and XIX (Medicaid) of the Social Security Act	Medicare provided health insurance for persons over the age of 65 who were receiving Social Security benefits. • Part A covered hospitalization. • Part B covered physicians' and outpatient services, after the beneficiary met a yearly deductible. Medicaid provided health care for families receiving Aid to Families with Dependent Children (AFDC). States had discretion over administering and determining program eligibility.
1972	President Nixon signed Public Law 92-603, which amended Medicare	The act expanded Medicare coverage to disabled people who had been receiving Social Security benefits for at least two years and to people with serious kidney disease.
1973	President Nixon signed the Health Maintenance Organizations Act	The act promoted health maintenance organizations (HMOs) over fee-for-service plans: • Eliminated state laws that prohibited HMOs. • Provided subsidies to establish "federally qualified" HMOs. • Created standards for HMOs (must be nonprofit, provide a certain level of care, and charge all members the same premium). • Required employers who offered health insurance to offer an HMO. • Allowed HMOs to adopt a variety of organizational structures.
1985	President Reagan signed the Consolidated Omnibus Budget Reconciliation Act (COBRA)	COBRA allowed employees to continue healthcare coverage if they were going to lose it due to job loss, death, or divorce of a family member, reduction in hours, or medical leave. The employee would pay both the employee and employer portions of the premium for 18 months to 36 months, depending on the qualifying event.
1996	President Clinton signed the Health Insurance Portability and Accountability Act (HIPAA)	HIPAA enabled workers to retain their health insurance after losing or changing jobs. It also limited the ability of insurance companies to exclude people with pre-existing conditions or charge them higher premiums for preexisting conditions or genetic predispositions.

(continued)

Table 8.1

Timeline of Health Care Legislation in the United States (*continued*)

Date	Legislation	Impact
		HIPAA also established national standards for the privacy and security of electronic health information. States could allow federal HIPAA regulations or adopt and enforce their own that would be at least as stringent as the federal legislation.
1997	President Clinton signed the Balanced Budget Act	The act created Title XXI of the Social Security Act, the State Children's Health Insurance Program (S-CHIP). It provided block grants for states to cover insurance for children who were not eligible for Medicaid but whose families earned less than 200 percent of the federal poverty line. The act also included changes to Medicare, formalizing Part C or Medicare Advantage.
2003	President Bush signed the Medicare Prescription Drug, Improvement and Modernization Act	The act allowed the participants in Medicare to select Part D for prescription coverage. It also made changes to Medicare Part B by charging higher premiums to higher-income beneficiaries and offered a tax exemption for health savings accounts (HSAs).
2010	President Obama signed the Patient Protection and Affordable Care Act (ACA or Obamacare)	The act expanded health insurance coverage through health insurance exchanges as well as through employer-provided plans. It required plans to provide coverage for dependent children to age 26 and prevented them from denying coverage or charging more for pre-existing conditions. The act also provided subsidies and tax credits, and allowed for and expansion of Medicaid to cover low-income childless adults. The act specified minimum mandatory coverage for • Ambulatory patient services. • Emergency services. • Hospitalization. • Maternity and newborn care. • Mental health and substance abuse disorder services, including behavioral health treatment. • Prescription drugs.

Table 8.1

Timeline of Health Care Legislation in the United States (*continued*)

Date	Legislation	Impact
		• Rehabilitative (regaining skills lost due to illness or injury) and habilitative services and devices (helping gain skills previously not attainable). • Laboratory services. • Preventive and wellness services and chronic disease management. • Pediatric services, including oral and vision care. The act gave states the option of creating a Basic Health Program (BHP) for both citizens and lawfully-residing noncitizens who do not qualify for other coverage and have an income between 133 percent and 200 percent of the federal poverty level. Minnesota and New York implemented BHPs beginning in 2015.

health care and providing more services was often associated with worse outcomes than providing less intensive care for lower costs. Using Medicare and Medicaid data, the Dartmouth Atlas Project[21] now publishes data on variations in medical resource use throughout the United States. It provides data by hospital, particularly on intensity of care near the end of life. This information is necessary for physicians to see how overtreatment does not equate with better outcomes. It also shows where intensive care unit stays are excessive and how hospice care is important for reducing interventions that are costly yet futile. Indeed, for the first time many physicians asked themselves whether the number of pain-free days is not just as important as how long their patients live—whether quality of life is at least as important as length of life.

In New Jersey, patients now have the option to control their treatments near the end of life. In December 2011, Governor Christie signed New Jersey's Practitioner Orders for Life-Sustaining Treatment (POLST) law to help patients and their families with end-of-life planning.[22] Unlike an advance directive, which is often disregarded by first responders or hospital staff who are trained to save lives, the POLST form is completed by a patient jointly with a physician, physician assistant, or advance practice nurse. It expresses the patient's goals for care and his or her medical preferences. A completed POLST form is treated as a medical order, and it becomes a part of the patient's medical record. The form is valid in all healthcare settings, following the patient from one healthcare setting to another, including hospital, nursing home, or hospice.

Findings such as those published by the Dartmouth Atlas Project led to the creation of a new field: outcomes research. Proponents of outcomes research have called for a major shift in the way health care is measured. For example, should we not measure the cost-effectiveness of conservative versus aggressive treatments? Could outpatient treatments be as effective as inpatient ones? Is patient satisfaction important? Such questions began to identify additional shortfalls in healthcare practices, and these led to strategies for improvements in the quality of care. But improved care can only improve outcomes for those with access to that care. What about those without access? How can those disparities be addressed?

It is well established that lacking health insurance is associated with an increased risk of subsequent mortality.[23-25] The 1965 Medicare and Medicaid Acts provided access to health insurance for seniors and those below the poverty line, but it did not solve social determinants of poverty or address the problems the near poor had in securing access health care services for their high-risk groups. Yet the National Health Interview Survey reported that in 1980 12.5 percent of the population still had no health insurance. By 1990, that proportion increased to 16.6 percent.[10]

The reasons for the increase in the uninsured population included the fact that full-time jobs with health insurance were going overseas and many employers were shifting the costs for rapidly increasing premiums to their employees. Some employers ceased offering health insurance at all. Job loss and cost shifting meant that many Americans could no longer afford health insurance. For others, it meant becoming underinsured because policies no longer covered pre-existing medical conditions, required copayments and deductibles that caused delays in care, and blocked certain categories of benefits (e.g., mental health). Cost sharing was promoted as a way to reduce overutilization, but it masked the challenge of measuring how access to care was related to health outcomes. Without access, the uninsured were left to their own devices—either going without care or using emergency rooms when no other solution could be found. Even if they gained access through the emergency room, there was no guarantee they could gain access to medications or follow-up treatment.

A 1993 report by Millman for the National Academy of Sciences pointed out clearly that access to health care is only one of the factors that drive healthcare outcomes. Successful outcomes may fail for a number of reasons:

- The treatment is inappropriate for that patient.
- Some percentage of all disease processes may not respond to the appropriate treatment.
- The treatment is of questionable efficacy.
- The disease defeats the best that medical care can offer.
- The diagnostic and treatment skills of the provider are below acceptable standards.
- The patient does not follow the treatment regimen.[26]

In other words, even with the best treatment, good outcomes cannot be guaranteed.

What we can do, however, is to make sure that people have the opportunity for a good outcome. Millman argued that, rather than a focus on reducing immediate costs or improving underutilization for those who lack insurance, the goal should be to improve the quality of health care for all. As an example, he pointed out that an insured patient with complex problems requiring multiple services would benefit from adding a case manager (care coordinator). The poor and uninsured might require even more than that. They might require a case manager and a social worker who could combine health care with social services and who would follow up with the patient for personal health care.

For examples of how poverty, access to health care, and health outcomes are intertwined, consider the cases of Newark and Camden in New Jersey. Over the decades, both cities suffered from urban unrest, white flight to the suburbs, loss of manufacturing jobs, urban renewal that disrupted neighborhoods, and declining educational systems (see chapters 3, 5, and 6). Despite efforts to provide Medicare, Medicaid, Obamacare, and the State Children's Health Insurance Program (SCHIP), the differences in the proportion of the population under age 65 who were without health insurance remained stark in these cities compared with New Jersey as a whole (Table 8.2). Both cities have populations that are more Black and Brown than the state as a whole, as well as more residents who are poor or disabled.

One of the most sensitive health outcome measures is the infant mortality rate (IMR). *Healthy People 2020* set the national IMR target at 6.0 deaths

Table 8.2

Estimated Select Demographic Measures for Camden, Newark, and the State of New Jersey, 2019

Measure	Camden	Newark	New Jersey
Total population	73,562	282,011	8,882,190
Population white, not Hispanic or Latino	23.5%	11.0%	54.6%
Persons in poverty	36.4%	27.4%	9.2%
Persons without health insurance < 65 years	12.7%	19.1%	9.2%
Persons with a disability < 65 years	15.1%	11.9%	6.5%

SOURCE: U.S. Census QuickFacts.[27]

per 1,000 live births. By 2018, the New Jersey IMR was among the lowest in the nation at 3.6 per 1,000 live births.[28] In Newark, however, the story was not so rosy. Roche et al.[29] examined birth and linked death certificate data from 2000 to 2006 by zip code for the greater Newark region. The IMRs for the zip codes in the region ranged from 4.3 to 16.6 per 1,000 live births. These findings were not surprising in that pregnant women who received no prenatal care had higher odds of infant mortality compared with women who received prenatal care. A bit more surprising was that maternal nativity and education were not significant predictors of outcome. The researchers found that zip codes with the lowest IMRs were outside the city proper; these places had the highest average family income, the lowest percentage of people living below the poverty level, and the lowest proportion of Black residents. The zip codes with the highest IMRs were within the Newark city limits; they had the lowest average family income, the highest percentage of people living below the poverty level, and the highest proportion of Black residents. They also had the largest proportion of uninsured. The study clearly demonstrated how the most sensitive health outcome, the IMR, is intertwined with both poverty and access to care.

Now consider Camden, a city that suffered from corruption so rampant that the state stripped the city government of most of its authority in 2002. In 2004 and 2005, Camden was identified as the number one most dangerous city in America. In 2012, the Federal Bureau of Investigation ranked Camden at 1 for violent crime among all cities with populations over 50,000. That meant that Camden in 2012 was more dangerous than Oakland, California, and Detroit and Flint, Michigan.[30] The conditions in Camden showed how crime, corruption, and poverty can be intertwined with health outcomes. In February 2001, a twenty-two-year-old Black Rutgers University student was shot several times, then was left lying in the street. After a police officer on the scene declared that the victim was unlikely to survive, no one even made an effort to save him. The police were just standing around, not even close to the body, when Jeffrey Brenner, a physician who lived a few houses away, became horrified by their lack of effort and began chest compression and rescue breathing for the victim himself. Although the student died, Brenner pursued his concerns with the police and wound up serving on a police reform commission in Camden as a citizen member.

The commission wanted computerized crime maps to help them study the problem of crime throughout the city, but the police refused to create them. This led Brenner to create his own maps from emergency room data, bolstered by hospital billing data. Although the commission was eventually disbanded, the new data set Brenner had created was an eye opener. He found that he could now track ambulance calls, locate addresses that generated high medical costs, and, with permission, even identify the individuals who cycled in and out of the hospital with repeat admissions. In fact, Brenner's effort to map hotspots of crime led him in an entirely different direction; he found that just 1 percent of the 100,000 people who made use of Camden's medical facilities accounted for 30 percent of its costs.[31] Readers who wish to view an excellent short documentary on Brenner's experience and his findings should watch the PBS *Frontline* episode, "Dr. Hotspot."[32]

After Brenner's identification of "super-utilizers" of health care, the Camden Coalition enrolled these high-cost patients into a coordinated outpatient care system that included a team of nurses, social workers, and community health workers. Did the coordinated care system work? The answer here is *perhaps*.[33] But long before the program was evaluated through a randomized clinical trial, the strategy was adopted by hospitals and third-party payers across the nation in an attempt to reduce direct healthcare costs. Since then, the strategy has expanded in scope, particularly because the ACA carries penalties for avoidable readmissions. For instance, if you have health insurance, you may now find that a nurse or care coordinator will call you to remind you to get a mammogram, have your blood pressure checked, or reorder your medications. After you have had a surgical procedure, you are likely to receive a call from a nurse to check on how you are doing and be sure you are following your discharge instructions.

Such proactive efforts may seem intrusive to some, but they do preempt some costly hospitalizations. They also have been shown to improve both clinical outcomes and patient satisfaction.[34,35] Once Medicare began offering billing codes for chronic care management,[36] private insurers followed suit and most now cover coordinated care. The problem remains, however, for those who are uninsured. In Camden, that number remains at almost 13 percent of the population under age sixty-five as of 2019.[37]

The problems of crime and corruption in Camden grew as a result of industrial decay, joblessness, and the flight of those who could afford to leave the city (see chapters 3 and 6). The city's estimated population in 2020 was young, with about 31 percent under the age of eighteen years. It was also more Black and Brown than the state as a whole, with 41 percent Black and 51 percent Latino residents.[27] Camden stands as an exemplar for how crime, corruption, and poverty impact health through social determinant problems (see chapter 5). But the efforts in Camden lit a spark that helped shift the health care industry into providing coordinated health care that links to social services. This shift is laudable for health outcomes, but it has not been effective in lowering the continued rise in rates for health insurance premiums. Indeed, the Centers for Medicare & Medicaid Services projects national health spending will increase at an average rate of 5.5 percent each year to 2027, eventually reaching $6 trillion dollars.[38]

We have highlighted Camden and Newark in this chapter, but New Jersey's other historically poor and minority cities also struggle with health disparities and upstream factor influences. For more examples of these circumstances, see the age-adjusted death rates, COVID-19 outcomes, and vaccination rates for Atlantic City, Passaic, Paterson, and Trenton in chapter 5.

More Attempts to Manage Care and Lower Costs

At the beginning of the 1980s, there were about 7,000 active hospitals in the United States. By 2020, there were about 1,000 fewer of them.[39] Hospitals faced pressures to close excess beds and reduce the number of employees.[40] At the same time, a new disease challenged existing healthcare resources. By June 1990, 139,765 people in the United States had human immunodeficiency virus/acquired immunodeficiency syndrome, and the cases had a 60 percent mortality rate (see chapter 5). Fully 44 million Americans, 16 percent of the population, had no health insurance at all.[41] It was clear that the next few decades would require radical changes if the health-care system was to stay afloat.

Improvements in both hardware and software in the 1990s allowed for bet-ter computerized record-keeping of diseases, treatments, and costs. State and national disease registries, electronic medical records, and the tracking of treatment outcomes and patient satisfaction were scrutinized by both hospi-tals and insurers. Simply put, the world entered the era of big data. Big data put big change into the wind as health care moved toward "evidence-based practice"[42] for both clinicians[43] and health administrators.[44] Hospitals posted data on private physicians to increase peer pressure on those who "churned" patients by ordering consults and additional testing to increase their own charges. Full-time hospitalists were hired to control and reduce lengths of stay and to serve as a check on abuses of services by private physicians. Best prac-tices were promulgated to reduce avoidable risks and lessen readmissions.

Small hospitals closed,[45,46] or they were gobbled up by consolidations into hospital systems with more efficient purchasing power and control of operations.[47-49] In May 2021, the American Hospital Association listed 5,141 hospitals in the United States, of which 3,453 were in a system.[50] New Jersey had seventy-one acute care hospitals, of which fifty-six were in a system. The number of in-system hospitals in the state is likely to further increase; at the time of this writing several others were currently in negotia-tions. Although being in a system increases a facility's power to negotiate higher reimbursement rates and it should improve patient safety through the sharing of best practices, it also means facilities lose their autonomy.

Most hospitals in the United States (57 percent) are not-for-profit com-munity hospitals. The rest are for-profit (24 percent) or government-owned (19 percent).[51] By 2021 in New Jersey, eleven of the seventy-one acute care hospitals in the state were listed as for-profit (15 percent). How the for-profit status of hospitals will play out for healthcare costs, particularly given the challenges of caring for COVID patients and burned out hospital staff, has yet to be determined.

Select medical services in hospitals also consolidated into centers that mar-keted their expertise to treat complex cases (e.g., cancer,[51] stroke,[52] and trauma centers[53]). A Google search in 2021 listed twenty cancer centers, twenty trauma centers, and twenty stroke centers in New Jersey—places where resi-dents could get primary treatment. Another search, however, showed that some institutions are marketing the claim to be a center without the appropriate designation from either the state or a national organization.

For example, the designation as a comprehensive cancer center means that the National Cancer Institute (NCI) has determined that the institution has met its standard for cancer prevention, clinical services, and research.[54] At the time of this writing, only one NCI-designated comprehensive cancer center exists in New Jersey, the Rutgers Cancer Institute in New Brunswick.

A search for comprehensive stroke centers—a certification given by both the Joint Commission[55] and the state of New Jersey[56]—showed eight and thirteen New Jersey hospitals, respectively (Table 8.3). In its criteria for certification as a comprehensive stroke center, the Joint Commission (a partnership between the American Heart Association and the American Stroke Association) requires the availability of advanced imaging techniques along with 24/7 availability of personnel trained in vascular neurology, neurosurgery, and endovascular procedures.

A search for verified trauma centers (certified by the American College of Surgeons[57]) showed four NJ hospitals providing level I services and another six providing level II (Table 8.3). A level I trauma center can provide services that cover all aspects of an injury, from prevention to rehabilitation. These include twenty-four-hour in-house coverage by general surgeons and prompt availability of care for orthopedic surgery, neurosurgery, anesthesiology, emergency medicine, radiology, internal medicine, plastic surgery with oral and maxillofacial treatment, pediatric and critical care, and a minimum annual volume of severely injured patients. A level II trauma center can initiate definitive care for all injured patients but may refer tertiary care needs to a level I trauma center. Trauma centers are marked with standardized road signs across the country, and many have heliports.

Similarly, many U.S. hospitals now have a dedicated a floor or wing that is marketed as a children's hospital. Cassimir[58] states there are now more than 250 children's hospitals in the United States and that pediatric departments in general hospitals are no longer the standard of care. A children's hospital provides pediatric-trained surgeons, anesthetists, radiologists, and allied health professionals as well as appropriately-sized machines for diagnosis and treatment in order to obtain the best outcomes. Given that one in six discharges from American hospitals in 2012 were of children under the age of eighteen years and the majority of these stays were for infants, this is a segment of the population hospitals cannot ignore. In the United States, half of all the care provided in children's hospitals goes to disadvantaged children, and 6 percent of these cases are medically complex, requiring ongoing care for serious, long-term conditions. Thus, the cost of care is

Table 8.3

Centers for Cancer, Stroke, and Trauma in New Jersey, 2021

Designation	Institution
Comprehensive Cancers Centers	• Rutgers Cancer Institute of New Jersey, New Brunswick
Comprehensive Stroke Centers*	• AtlanticCare Regional Medical Center, Atlantic City • Capital Health System at Fuld, Trenton* • Community Hospital Group, Inc., Edison • Cooper Health System, Camden • Hackensack University Medical Center, Hackensack • Jersey Shore Medical Center, Neptune • Kennedy University Hospital, Washington Township* • Morristown Memorial Hospital, Morristown* • Overlook Hospital, Summit • Robert Wood Johnson University Hospital, New Brunswick • St. Barnabas Medical Center, Newark* • St. Joseph's Medical Center* • University Hospital, Newark • Valley Hospital, Ridgewood*
Verified Level I Trauma Centers	• Cooper University Health Care, Camden • Morristown Medical Center, Morristown • New Jersey Trauma Center at the University Hospital, Newark • Robert Wood Johnson University Hospital, New Brunswick
Verified Level II Trauma Centers	• AtlantiCare Regional Medical Center, Atlantic City • Capital Health Regional Medical Center, Trenton • Hackensack University Medical Center, Hackensack • Jersey City Medical Center, Jersey City • Jersey Shore University Medical Center, Neptune • St Joseph's Regional Medical Center, Paterson

*Certified by the New Jersey Department of Health only.

NOTE: The listings reflect the names of institutions as presented by accrediting body documents. The names of the institutions may have changed since publication.

SOURCE: American College of Surgeons,[57] Joint Commission,[55] National Cancer Institute,[54] and the New Jersey Department of Health.[56]

greater for pediatric patients than for adults, albeit the reimbursements are lower. Because pediatric inpatient care is not profitable, hospitals are moving toward reducing pediatric length of stays whenever possible, and they are developing dedicated outpatient facilities for children with services that involve family members in care.

As inpatient services across the nation were consolidating, outpatient services were becoming more widely distributed. Minute clinics popped up to provide a quick, easy way for people who feel sick (but not sick enough to go to an emergency department) to seek medical treatment without having to wait for a doctor's appointment.[59,60] Vaccine programs became widely available at pharmacies, including those located within big box stores and supermarkets, again providing a service outside a doctor's office or clinic appointment.[61] When vaccines became available for COVID-19, countless locations and several mega and pop-up sites were established to handle the volume. The use of telemedicine to provide clinical services and telehealth to provide clinical, healthcare training, public health, and administrative services also began to rise in the 2000s as more patients and their providers had access to better internet services.

Beginning with providing emergency and other medical services to remote areas (e.g., northern Alaska or the base of the Grand Canyon), telemedicine became increasingly important to Americans who did have access to medical care but preferred remote care options. For example, Reed and colleagues[62] completed a cross-sectional study of patients who scheduled a primary care visit in northern California between January 2016 and May 2018. Routine physicals were excluded because they were ineligible for telemedicine coverage. More than 2 million primary care visits were scheduled by more than 1 million patients during this period. Of those visits, 86 percent were in-office, and 14 percent were via telemedicine, 7 percent of which were by video. Patients over age sixty-five years of age were less likely to choose telemedicine compared with those aged eighteen to forty-four. Uptake of telemedicine visits was associated with living in a neighborhood with high rates of residential internet access but barriers to inpatient visits (such as lengthy transportation time or a lack of access to free parking at the healthcare facility). Of interest is that female patients were more likely than male patients to choose telemedicine, and Black patients were more likely to choose both phone and video visits than any other race/ethnicity. The study noted the opportunities their findings presented for engaging more non-white patients, those with mobile technology, and those who face barriers to in-person visits in telemedicine.

The COVID-19 pandemic challenged the existing healthcare system beyond the imaginable. Necessity required practitioners to radically alter how they provided care to their patients, and many offices without sufficient staff and personal protective equipment simply shut down. Medical centers quickly adopted telemedicine and virtual care in order to deliver timely care while minimizing exposure for both practitioners and patients. Medicare, Medicaid, and private insurers began to cover more than eighty new services via telemedicine.[63,64] The AMA also reported that physicians now see fifty to 175 times the number of patients via telehealth than they did before the pandemic.[65] How did this happen?

Wosik et al.[66] described the shift to telehealth once the pandemic began. As they explain, changes first occurred in outpatient demand (phase 1), then during the hospital surge (phase 2), followed by the postpandemic recovery period (phase 3). At the beginning of phase 1, there was limited demand for outpatient telehealth visits for either e-consults or urgent care. Once the stay-at-home orders occurred, the demand for both telephone and video visits rapidly increased, and the supply expanded to meet the need. As social distancing relaxed, the demand for outpatient telehealth lessened somewhat, but it remained at a relatively high rate.

At the beginning of phase 2, there was limited use of inpatient telehealth, but after the stay-at-home orders began the demand for virtual consults increased (i.e., TeleICU). Once social distancing requirements were relaxed, the demand for inpatient telehealth decreased somewhat; but because the services had become billable, they stabilized at a new high-normal. Phase 3 dealt with the needs of patients who had deferred seeking diagnosis and treatment for serious conditions, including surgeries, due to the stay-at-home order. Once the social distancing requirement was relaxed, there was a surge for services to address both acute and chronic care complications, services that could not be provided remotely.

Given that there is now a new demand for telemedicine, and given that these services are now billable, what is in store for the future? Bestsennyy et al.[67] have calculated that adopting various telehealth models could save up to $250 billion of current U.S. healthcare spending. Telehealth services could include

1   On-demand virtual urgent care as an alternative to lesser acuity emergency department visits, urgent care visits, and after-hours consultations.

2 Virtual office visits with an established provider for consults that do not require physical examinations or concurrent procedures.

3 Near-virtual office visits that combine virtual access to physician consults with "near home" in-person sites for testing and immunizations.

4 Virtual home health services, including remote monitoring and digital patient engagement tools (e.g., portions of evaluations, patient and care giver education, physical therapy, occupational therapy, and speech therapy).

5 Tech-enabled home medication administration (e.g., infusible and injectable drugs administered in the home) after patient or care-giver education and with telehealth oversight of staff.

These researchers estimate that approximately 20 percent of all emergency room visits could be avoided via virtual urgent care, 24 percent of office visits could be delivered virtually, and an additional 9 percent could be delivered "near-virtually." Furthermore, up to 35 percent of regular home health attendant services could be virtualized, and 2 percent of all outpatient volume could be shifted to the home setting (with tech-enabled medication administration).

Upstream Responses to Health Care

The future of health care seems to be moving toward newer treatments, newer technologies, and more online and distributed services, factors that can improve healthcare outcomes for patients but hold little promise for cost containment. Providing access to health insurance through the ACA is one approach that increased the focus on outcomes and is moving the system farther from fee-for-service toward pay-for-performance (a value-based system that ties reimbursement to metric-driven outcomes, proven best practices, and patient satisfaction).[68] The success of the ACA can also be touted because New Jersey now has 800,000 residents covered by the program, a record-low uninsured rate for the state.[69] Prevention programs are now embraced by the healthcare community as important for reducing risk for individuals. But what if we used a different approach to prevention rather than a medical one?

Chapter 1 defined upstream factors as the social-structural influences on population health and health systems, including government policies, as well as the social, physical, economic, and environmental factors that determine health. We can trace the beginning of interest in upstream factors to the Healthy Cities movement, an idea promoted in the mid-1980s during an International Conference on Health Promotion in Toronto, Canada. The idea spread to the United States in the late 1980s where it expanded to the Healthy Communities movement, an idea championed by public health rather than the healthcare community.[70]

By the late 1990s, federal agencies, national nonprofits, health foundations, and a few healthcare systems had an interest in the Healthy Communities concept; some launched initiatives of varying scales. For instance, in 2001, the National Association of County and City Health Officials in cooperation with the Public Health Practice Program Office at Centers for Disease Control and Prevention (CDC) launched Mobilizing for Action through Planning and Partnerships (MAPP). MAPP is a community-driven strategic planning process for community health improvement. The process results in a community health assessment (CHA) that identifies community problems and assets, as well as measuring how well a public health system is fulfilling its function.[71] CHAs are also used to create community health improvement plans (CHIPs), which identify priority issues, set measurable targets for health improvement, and develop strategies for action that hopefully involve many community organizations.

In the first decade of 2000, the Robert Wood Johnson Foundation (RWJF) and health systems such as Kaiser Permanente established grant programs to nurture collaborations among the community development, public health, and healthcare sectors.[72] The American Public Health Association and the American Planning Association created toolboxes and guidelines for practice for their members, but some in the healthcare sector were dragging their heels. The ACA of 2010 changed that. It forced collaborations across the three sectors by requiring hospitals to engage with and reinvest in the communities they serve.[73]

The ACA requires tax-exempt hospitals to create a community health needs assessment (CHNA) every three years. Failure to compete a mandated CHNA carries a severe penalty: hospitals could lose their tax-exempt status under section 501 of the tax code and be penalized with up to $50,000 in fines for each year the hospital is out of compliance.[74] CHNAs must be developed with community stakeholders and must include:

- A demographic assessment of the community the hospital serves.
- A needs assessment of perceived community healthcare issues.

- A quantitative analysis of actual community healthcare issues.
- Appraisal of current efforts to address the identified healthcare issues.
- A three-year plan for the hospital and the community to collectively address any remaining issues.

CHIPs ensure collaboration across sectors as they lay out long-term, systematic efforts to address community health problems. CHAs are used by public health agencies and CHNAs are used by hospitals, but CHIPs are used by health, education, and human service agencies along with community partners to set priorities and target resources. CHIPs define a vision for community health but only with input from that same community.[75] Readers interested in reviewing all current CHAs, CHNAs, and CHIPs in New Jersey can find them posted on the Healthy New Jersey website.[75] They offer a different perspective about organizing and delivering health care than has been the history in the United States.

In 2014, RWJF funded the Build Healthy Places Network[76] to change the way neighborhoods are revitalized by integrating health and community development. The Plan 4 Health project was also funded by CDC as a three-year project to strengthen the connection between the planning and public health professions.[77] A 2021 a Google search for "Healthy Communities" still brings the RWJF website to the top of the results, reminding those seeking foundation funding that the built environment, public and community health, health disparities, and the social determinants of health are upstream factors that can change the overall health of the population. Simply focusing on the healthcare sector will not make the changes we need to bring down healthcare costs and improve health outcomes.

Although the United States does not have a single healthcare system, we are certainly moving toward several consolidated ones, and COVID-19 may have given that trend a shove. Abelson[78] writes that the pandemic barely dented the financial outlook for some major healthcare networks. The $178 billion Provider Relief Fund passed by Congress to alleviate stresses on hospitals due to the pandemic allocated the bulk of the money to the wealthiest hospital systems, placing no limits on the use of the funds. Thus, many systems used the funding for mergers and acquisitions, acquiring weaker hospitals and physician practices. In other words, we now have larger hospital systems with more power than before the pandemic.

This returns us to the discussion of Health in All Policies (chapter 1) and our explanation about how federal and state policies affect more than one sector. During the pandemic, the healthcare sector took the brunt of emergency visits and hospitalizations; the public health sector was charged with health education and immunizations; and the community development sector took on food distribution and the many problems associated with quarantine. Federal policy allowed new vaccines to be used under U.S. Food and Drug Administration (FDA) emergency use authorization. State policies defined vaccine distribution and mask requirements, along with school and business closures. Communities deployed police, fire, school, and volunteer community assets. While some may question the effectiveness of the U.S. response to the pandemic, the interconnectedness of these sectors became clear. We need the cooperation of all of the sectors to improve health for all.

References

1 Dawidziak M. Legendary CBS anchor Walter Cronkite dies at 92. *Cleveland Plain Dealer/Associated Press*, July 18, 2009. https://www.cleveland.com/nation/2009/07/walter_cronkite_dies_at_92_rep.html
2 Cronin JW, Odoroff ME. *Hospital Beds in the United States, 1951.* Washington, DC: U.S. Public Health Service; 1952.
3 Health Resources & Services Administration. Hill-Burton Free and Reduced-Cost Health Care. Updated March 2022. https://www.hrsa.gov/get-health-care/affordable/hill-burton/index.html
4 Health Resources & Services Administration. Hill-Burton facilities obligated to provide free or reduced-cost health care. Updated March 2022. https://www.hrsa.gov/get-health-care/affordable/hill-burton/facilities.html
5 2013 New Jersey Revised Statutes Title 26—Health and Vital Statistics Section 26: 2H-18.64—Denial of admission on ability to pay; penalty. *Justia US Law.* https://law.justia.com/codes/new-jersey/2013/title-26/section-26-2h-18.64/
6 Volpp KG, Siegel B. New Jersey: Long-term experience with all-payer state rate setting. *Health Aff.* 1993;12(2):59–65. doi:10.1377/hlthaff.12.2.59
7 New Jersey Department of Health. Charity Care—New Jersey Hospital Care Payment Assistance Program: Regulations and Public Notices. Accessed May 28, 2021. https://www.nj.gov/health/charitycare/regs-public-notices/
8 Zibulewsky J. The Emergency Medical Treatment and Active Labor Act (EMTALA): what it is and what it means for physicians. *Baylor Univ Med Cent Proc.* 2001;14(4):339–346. doi:10.1080/08998280.2001.11927785
9 New Jersey Hospital Association. N.J.A.C. 8:43G Subchapter 12—Emergency Department and Trauma Services EMTALA—CMS Final Rule 489.20(1). March 10, 2011. https://www.njacep.org/Portals/0/Documents/110309_ED_Regs.pdf
10 *Healthcare Crisis:* healthcare timeline. PBS, August 2000. https://www.pbs.org/healthcarecrisis/history.htm
11 Medicare and Medicaid. LBJ Presidential Library, December 2017. https://web.archive.org/web/20210730225434/http://www.lbjlibrary.org/press/media-kit/medicare-and-medicaid

12 Social Security Administration. Social Security history: Medicare is signed into law. n.d. https://www.ssa.gov/history/lbjsm.html

13 Arrow KJ. Uncertainty and the welfare economics of medical care. *Am Econ Rev.* 1963;53(5):941–973. https://www.jstor.org/stable/1812044

14 Heiser SS. The majority of U.S. medical students are women, new data show. Association of American Medical Colleges press release. December 9, 2019. https://www.aamc.org/news-insights/press-releases/majority-us-medical-students -are-women-new-data-show

15 Are female doctors paid less? See the gap, in 6 charts. *Advisory Board*, September 23, 2020. https://www.advisory.com/en/daily-briefing/2020/09/23/female-compensation

16 Congress passes historic GME expansion. AAMC. December 23, 2020. https:// www.aamc.org/advocacy-policy/washington-highlights/congress-passes-historic -gme-expansion

17 Tobias M. Comparing administrative costs for private insurance and Medicare. *PolitiFact*, September 20, 2017. https://www.politifact.com/factchecks/2017/sep /20/bernie-sanders/comparing-administrative-costs-private-insurance-a/

18 Hsiao WC, Sapolsky HM, Dunn DL, Weiner SL. Lessons of the New Jersey DRG payment system. *Health Aff (Millwood)*. 1986;5(2):32–45. doi:10.1377/ hlthaff.5.2.32

19 Dickerson PS. Health care reform in New Jersey. In: Abbott T III, ed. *Health Care Policy and Regulation*. New York: Springer Science; 2011:93–95.

20 Wennberg J, Gittelsohn A. Small area variations in health care delivery. *Science.* 1973;182(4117):1102–1108. doi:10.1126/science.182.4117.1102

21 The Dartmouth Atlas Project. *The Dartmouth Atlas of Health Care*. Lebanon, NH: Trustees of Dartmouth College; updated 2019. https://www.dartmout hatlas.org/

22 New Jersey Department of Health. Practitioner Orders for Life-Sustaining Treatment (POLST). Updated January 31, 2022. https://www.state.nj.us/health /advancedirective/polst/

23 Kronick R. Health insurance coverage and mortality revisited. *Health Serv Res.* 2009;44(4):1211–1231. doi:10.1111/j.1475-6773.2009.00973.x

24 Wilper AP, Woolhandler S, Lasser KE, et al. Health insurance and mortality in US adults. *Am J Public Health*. 2009;99(12):2289–2295. doi:10.2105/AJPH.2008 .157685

25 Kilbourne AM. Care without coverage: too little, too late. *J Natl Med Assoc.* 2005;97(11):1578. https://www.ncbi.nlm.nih.gov/pmc/articles/PMC2594911/

26 Institute of Medicine, Committee on Monitoring Access to Personal Health Care Services. *Access to Health Care in America*. Washington, DC: National Academies Press; 1993. doi:10.17226/2009

27 U.S. Census Bureau. QuickFacts: United States. Accessed May 5, 2021. https:// www.census.gov/quickfacts/fact/table/US/PST040219

28 New Jersey State Health Assessment Data. Center for Health Statistics. Accessed May 5, 2021. https://web.archive.org/web/20061109205526/http://njshad.doh .state.nj.us/welcome.html

29 Roche NE, Abdul-Hakeem F, Davidow AL, et al. The epidemiology of infant mortality in the greater Newark, New Jersey area: a new look at an old problem. *J Natl Med Assoc.* 2016;108(1):45–53. doi:10.1016/j.jnma.2015.12.007

30 Why is Camden consistently ranked #1 for crime in America? Lombardo Law Group, n.d. Accessed May 5, 2021. https://www.lombardolawoffices.com/why-is-camden-consistently-ranked-1-for-crime-in-america/

31 Gawande A. Finding medicine's hot spots. *New Yorker*, January 16, 2021. https://www.newyorker.com/magazine/2011/01/24/the-hot-spotters

32 Doctor Hotspot, *Frontline*, Season 2011, Episode 12, July 26, 2011. https://www.pbs.org/video/frontline-doctor-hotspot/

33 Finkelstein A, Zhou A, Taubman S, Doyle J. Health care hotspotting—a randomized, controlled trial. *N Engl J Med*. 2020;382(2):152–162. doi:10.1056/nejmsa1906848

34 Baxter S, Johnson M, Chambers D, et al. The effects of integrated care: a systematic review of UK and international evidence. *BMC Health Serv Res*. 2018;18:350. doi:10.1186/s12913-018-3161-3

35 Williams MD, Asiedu GB, Finnie D, et al. Sustainable care coordination: a qualitative study of primary care provider, administrator, and insurer perspectives. *BMC Health Serv Res*. 2019;19(1):1–10. doi:10.1186/s12913-019-3916-5

36 Centers for Medicare & Medicaid Services. Medicare Program; Revisions to Payment Policies Under the Physician Fee Schedule and Other Revisions to Part B for CY 2017; Medicare Advantage Bid Pricing Data Release; Medicare Advantage and Part D Medical Loss Ratio Data Release; Medicare Advantage Provider Network Requirements; Expansion of Medicare Diabetes Prevention Program Model; Medicare Shared Savings Program Requirements. Final rule. *Fed Regist*. 2016;81(220):80170–80562. https://www.govinfo.gov/content/pkg/FR-2016-11-15/pdf/2016-26668.pdf

37 U.S. Census Bureau. QuickFacts: Camden City, New Jersey. Accessed May 27, 2021. https://www.census.gov/quickfacts/fact/table/camdencitynewjersey/HEA775219

38 Centers for Medicare & Medicaid Services. National health expenditure projections 2018–2027 forecast summary. February 18, 2019. https://www.cms.gov/Research-Statistics-Data-and-Systems/Statistics-Trends-and-Reports/NationalHealthExpendData/Downloads/ForecastSummary.pdf

39 How many hospitals are in the US? *Definitive Healthcare Blog*, March 2, 2022. https://blog.definitivehc.com/how-many-hospitals-are-in-the-us

40 Wennberg JE. Wennberg: administrators must pursue policies that reduce excess beds, employees. *Heal Manag Q*. December 1984:6–7.

41 A Science Odyssey, People and Discoveries: AIDS is officially recognized. *PBS*, 1998. https://www.pbs.org/wgbh/aso/databank/entries/dm81ai.html

42 Agency for Healthcare Research and Quality. Evidence-based practice. n.d. Accessed May 7, 2021. https://www.ahrq.gov/topics/evidence-based-practice.html

43 Sackett D, Straus S, Richardson W, et al. *Evidence-Based Medicine: How to Practice and Teach EBM*. 2nd ed. Edinburgh: Churchill Livingstone; 2000.

44 Houser J, Oman KS. *Evidence-Based Practice: An Implementation Guide for Healthcare Organizations*. Burlington, MA: Jones and Bartlett Learning; 2011.

45 Mullner RM, Rydman RJ, Whiteis DG, Rich RF. Rural community hospitals and factors correlated with their risk of closing. *Public Health Rep*. 1989;104(4):315–325.

46 Lynch JR, Ozcan YA. Hospital closure: an efficiency analysis. *Hosp Health Serv Admin*. 1994;39(2):205–220.

47 Beaulieu ND, Dafny LS, Landon BE, et al. Changes in quality of care after hospital mergers and acquisitions. *N Engl J Med.* 2020;382(1):51–59. doi:10.1056/NEJMsa1901383

48 McCue MJ, Thompson JM, Kim TH. Hospital acquisitions before healthcare reform. *J Healthc Manag.* 2015;60(3):186–203. doi:10.1097/00115514-201505000-00007

49 Harrison TD. Consolidations and closures: an empirical analysis of exits from the hospital industry. *Health Econ.* 2007;16(5):457–474. doi:10.1002/hec.1174

50 American Hospital Association. Fast facts on U.S. hospitals. January 2021. https://www.aha.org/system/files/media/file/2021/01/Fast-Facts-Hospitals-Infographic-2021-jan21.pdf

51 National Cancer Institute. Find an NCI-designated cancer center. n.d. Accessed May 7, 2021. https://www.cancer.gov/research/infrastructure/cancer-centers/find

52 Schwamm LH, Pancioli A, Acker JE, et al. Recommendations for the establishment of stroke systems of care: recommendations from the American Stroke Association's Task Force on the Development of Stroke Systems. *Stroke.* 2005;36(3):690–703. doi:10.1161/01.STR.0000158165.42884.4F

53 American Trauma Society. Trauma center levels explained. n.d. Accessed April 28, 2021. https://www.amtrauma.org/page/traumalevels

54 National Cancer Institute. NCI-designated cancer centers. Updated June 24, 2019. https://www.cancer.gov/research/infrastructure/cancer-centers

55 The Joint Commission. Certification Data Download: Download Certification and Verification Data. QualityCheck.org. Accessed May 8, 2021. https://www.qualitycheck.org/data-download/certification-data-download/

56 New Jersey Department of Health, Office of Health Care Quality Assessment. Designated center hospitals by county: stroke services. Updated June 28, 2018. https://www.state.nj.us/health/healthcarequality/stroke/ctrhospitals_county.shtml

57 American College of Surgeons. Trauma centers, n.d. Accessed May 8, 2021. https://www.facs.org/search/trauma-centers?state=NJ&distance=100&n=50

58 Casimir G. Why children's hospitals are unique and so essential. *Front Pediatr.* 2019;7:305. doi:10.3389/fped.2019.00305

59 Mehrotra A, Wang MC, Lave JR, Adams JL, McGlynn EA. Retail clinics, primary care physicians, and emergency departments: a comparison of patients' visits. *Health Aff (Millwood).* 2008;27(5):1272–1282. doi:10.1377/hlthaff.27.5.1272

60 Mehrotra A, Liu H, Adams JL, et al. Comparing costs and quality of care at retail clinics with that of other medical settings for 3 common illnesses. *Ann Intern Med.* 2009;151(5):321–328. doi:10.7326/0003-4819-151-5-200909010-00006

61 Burson RC, Buttenheim AM, Armstrong A, Feemster KA. Community pharmacies as sites of adult vaccination: a systematic review. *Hum Vaccin Immunother.* 2016;12(12):3146–3159. doi:10.1080/21645515.2016.1215393

62 Reed ME, Huang J, Graetz I, et al. Patient characteristics associated with choosing a telemedicine visit vs office visit with the same primary care clinicians. *JAMA Netw Open.* 2020;3(6):e205873–e205873. doi:10.1001/jamanetworkopen.2020.5873

63 Centers for Medicare & Medicaid Services. FAQs on availability and usage of telehealth services through private health insurance coverage in response to coronavirus disease 2019 (COVID-19). March 24, 2020. https://www.cms.gov/files/document/faqs-telehealth-covid-19.pdf

64 Centers for Medicare & Medicaid Services. Medicare telemedicine health care provider fact sheet. *CMS.gov Newsroom*, March 17, 2020. https://www.cms.gov/newsroom/fact-sheets/medicare-telemedicine-health-care-provider-fact-sheet

65 Henry TA. After COVID-19, $250 billion in care could shift to telehealth. *AMA*, June 18, 2020. https://www.ama-assn.org/practice-management/digital/after-covid-19-250-billion-care-could-shift-telehealth

66 Wosik J, Fudim M, Cameron B, et al. Telehealth transformation: COVID-19 and the rise of virtual care. *J Am Med Informatics Assoc*. 2020;27(6):957–962. doi:10.1093/jamia/ocaa067

67 Bestsennyy O, Gilbert G, Harris A, Rost J. Telehealth: a post-COVID-19 reality? McKinsey & Company, July 9, 2021. https://www.mckinsey.com/industries/healthcare-systems-and-services/our-insights/telehealth-a-quarter-trillion-dollar-post-covid-19-reality

68 What is pay for performance in healthcare? *NEJM Catalyst*, March 1, 2018. https://catalyst.nejm.org/doi/full/10.1056/CAT.18.0245

69 New Jersey Hospital Association. Policy topics: healthcare coverage expansion. n.d. Accessed May 28, 2021. http://www.njha.com/policy-advocacy/policy-topics/healthcare-coverage-expansion/

70 Centers for Disease Control and Prevention. Healthy Communities Program (2008–2012). Updated March 7, 2017. https://www.cdc.gov/nccdphp/dch/programs/healthycommunitiesprogram/index.htm

71 Institute of Medicine, Committee on Assuring the Health of the Public in the 21st Century. *The Future of the Public's Health in the 21st Century*. Washington, DC: National Academies Press; 2003. doi:10.17226/10548

72 Robert Wood Johnson Foundation. Our focus areas: healthy communities. n.d. Accessed April 28, 2021. https://www.rwjf.org/en/our-focus-areas/focus-areas/healthy-communities.html

73 U.S. House of Representatives. Compilation of Patient Protection and Affordable Care Act [as amended through May 1, 2010]. June 9, 2010. https://www.hhs.gov/sites/default/files/ppacacon.pdf

74 Centers for Disease Control and Prevention. Community Health Assessments & Health Improvement Plans. Updated July 24, 2018. https://www.cdc.gov/publichealthgateway/cha/plan.html

75 State of New Jersey, Healthy New Jersey. Community plans, n.d. [2018]. Accessed May 8, 2021. https://www.nj.gov/health/healthynj/2030/community-plans/

76 Build Healthy Places Network. Accessed May 8, 2021. https://buildhealthyplaces.org/

77 Plan4Health. Accessed May 8, 2021. https://plan4health.us/

78 Abelson R. Big hospital chains get COVID aid, and buy up competitors. *New York Times*, May 21, 2020. https://www.nytimes.com/2021/05/21/health/covid-bailout-hospital-merger.html

Epilogue

————————————————————●

Confronting Challenges to
a Healthier New Jersey—
The Next 25 Years

> The future depends on what we do in
> the present.
> —Mahatma Gandhi

We began planning and then writing this book before the COVID-19 pandemic arrived in New Jersey. As we write this final chapter, the painful physical, social, and economic consequences of the virus underscore the absolute necessity of building a culture of health and pressing for Health in All Policies. Our American "can-do" attitude of fierce individualism and unbridled optimism helped us address the outbreak, but our plans were not always well-executed. The United States did lead the way in developing new vaccines, rapid testing, and drugs for treating COVID early, which are also prototypes for the future. This points out that while we need to maintain our individuality and can rely on innovation to some extent, we also need to work collectively to develop a healthy and sustainable future for us all. To do that, we need to face some very powerful social determinants of health.

Here we list seven of these determinants along with short summaries of the challenges they present. They may not be the only ones we should worry about, but we feel they require immediate attention and ongoing follow-up.

1 Pandemics and epidemics
2 Addictive behaviors
3 Coping with accelerated change and increased uncertainty
4 Cascading environmental threats
5 Growing disparities in economic, social, and political access
6 Demographic change
7 Politics, power, and hedgehog and fox strategies

Pandemics and Epidemics

The year 2020 was the year of COVID-19, and only a true optimist believed that the event would suddenly end by early 2021. We knew (1) there will be more cases, (2) the economy was wounded, and (3) our physical and social infrastructures need more help. Some schools reopened and stayed open. Sports opened up, but not everywhere. Vaccines were produced, but many questioned the side effects and refused the vaccine. Others refused to wear masks or practice social distancing. The politicization of the pandemic was remarkable, especially for those of us who generations earlier saw family members sicken or die from what are now vaccine-preventable diseases.

At the heart of why Health in All Policies and a culture of health are needed now more than ever is because another pandemic is sure to follow—we just do not know when. When author Michael Greenberg mentioned this possibility to a group of friends, the idea was greeted as if the devil had entered the room. The friends pointed out that the Spanish flu had occurred a century ago; if one of these deadly viruses only occurs every century, science will figure out a way of controlling it. Unfortunately, a more likely scenario is that another biological event will occur in the not-too-distant future. Our readers will recall that Hurricane Floyd was the most devastating tropical storm in New Jersey history when it struck in 1999. Then Irene in 2011 and Sandy in 2012 each broke previous records, and Ida followed them—showing us that these threats are sure to continue. Hence, the idea that there will not devastating events, including a pandemic as bad or even worse than COVID-19 in our future is wishful thinking.

Writing in 2005 about the severe acute respiratory syndrome (SARS) outbreak, Osterholm[1] described what needed to be done before the next novel virus hit. Middle East respiratory syndrome (MERS) appeared on the Arabian Peninsula in 2005, followed by the H1N1 flu in 2009, the Ebola epidemic in 2014, and the Zika virus epidemic in 2015–2016. Should COVID-19 have come as a surprise? The answer, he said, is no.

Osterholm and Olshaker[2] wrote another wake-up call in 2020, noting the deficiencies in our responses to epidemics and the lack of public-private leadership in preparing to handle them. Do we really want to control epidemics by waiting for two-thirds of the population to develop immunity through infection or for new vaccines to be developed? Osterholm and Olshaker[2] assert that COVID-19 is not even the "big one" and a future outbreak will be even larger. They call for developing a detailed plan for both short-term and long-term investments, and for actions we will need to take for the likely worse outbreak. Intersector planning must take place with medical suppliers, food producers and vendors, health care providers, drug and equipment producers, police, and other first responders, as well as those who transport goods. The need for ongoing research to develop drugs or other plans to control spread is also essential. Yet watching people refuse to wear masks, social distance, or otherwise refuse to practice risk-reducing behaviors has demonstrated the need for analyzing how to improve public participation and cooperation with public policy.

The United States has a history of not making long-term investments. We expect that within two years after the epidemic phase of this virus ends, we will see a precipitous drop in organizational preparedness and in funding for science and social science research. To avoid this distressing and predictable outcome, a program building a culture of health would raise the number of people willing to pressure government and businesses to stay prepared. A Health in All Policy process would connect COVID programs to other health-related programs that focus on social and environmental justice.

Addictive Behaviors

Almost everyone knows someone who smokes or vapes, or takes drugs, or drinks too much alcohol, many of whom started when they were young. These individuals may have faced immediate consequences for their actions, such as being involved in auto accidents or being arrested for substance abuse. If they did avoid the early consequences of their addictions, they may have suffered its longer-term effects, such as heart diseases and cancer. Unfortunately, much of the population has become inured to the health, economic, and social tolls associated with addictions and addictive behaviors.

International metrics tell us that Americans as a whole have become what Sachs calls a "mass addiction society."[3] Using disability-adjusted life years (DALYs) data for 2017, among 196 nations, the United States ranked first in cocaine, second in amphetamines and other drug use, and third in opioid-related DALYs. The nation also ranked fourth in mental disorders, fifth in anxiety illnesses, and eleventh in depressive disorders. There is no good news in these global comparisons, especially because the DALYs do not cover many other addictive issues facing the U.S. population. Almost half of all Americans have at least one addictive behavior,[3-7] including eating, exercise, and sex issues; use of digital media; gambling; obsessive shopping; and, of course, smoking. The "addictions without drugs," along with those related to legal and illegal substances, must all be addressed if we are to improve the health of the population over the next twenty-five years.[8]

We find it inconsistent that the federal government has launched major programs to stop drug smuggling into the United States but seems unable to curtail the overmarketing of some prescription drugs and addictive products that devastate populations. Critics say that elements of federal and some state government policies show the unwillingness of policy-makers to control the market-driven ambitions of businesses that profit from addictive behaviors. When combined with increasingly sophisticated marketing techniques and ease of access to addictive substances, the public is not being protected against their abuse.

The uncontrolled marketing of addictive products (alcohol, tobacco, vapes, gambling, video games and screens in general, along with prescription drugs) creates the need for counteractions. Sussman[6] and Sachs[3] offer suggestions, such as adding these addiction issues to school health curricula, and reaching out to community organizations and police and health departments to build cooperative outreach programs. We note that many of these have been tried with limited results—from community-based programs like DARE[9,10] to abstinence programs such as "Just Say No."[11] We also note the dearth of publicly financed programs to support psychological counseling for those suffering from addictions as well as the lack of support for programs to reduce the stigma attached to asking for mental health support.[12]

Rather than piloted programs with less than stellar results, a Health in All Policies decision-making component in federal and state legislation could begin to reframe the policy discussion. Instead of businesses simply being allowed to increase short-term profits, federal and state policies could substantially tax addictive products so they cover life-cycle costs or services like gambling recovery programs. This would create a measure of overall benefit to society and less incentive to market these addictions. Additionally, developing grassroots movements to create a culture of health at the local and state levels could possibly influence businesses to reduce promoting addictive behaviors or at least be honest about their destructive consequences.

Of all the challenges and trends we face, addictions remain a high priority because the United States lacks effective interventions. Local groups in progressive states can take the lead in pushing an addiction management agenda that includes anti-stigma campaigns and efforts to increase access to mental health services.

Coping with Accelerated Change and Increased Uncertainty

Globalization, automation, digitalization, pressure for opening or closing borders to immigrants, marketing of unprecedented amounts of information, and a warming climate are at the top of the list contributing to uncertainty and fear. Add to the mix a global pandemic, the decline of the economy, and moving education online causes many to feel that the unrelenting pace of change is overwhelming. Add to this the war in Eastern Europe, and most of us perceive a loss of order and often feel that we are living outside of our comfort zone. Some seek to restore a sense of familiarity by embracing addictive behaviors to ease their anxiety. Others view new ideas as a conspiracy to reduce their freedom of choice. They may even take positions that are counterproductive to improving health outcomes, such as refusing to wear masks or rejecting vaccinations.[13-18]

Globalization scares many people, and their fears are not entirely unfounded. Near the top of their fears is the integration of financial trade networks[18] fostered by Brazil, Russia, India, and China (BRIC countries), as well as Japan, the European Union, and others with increasing economic power.[19] Southern hemisphere nations no longer wish to serve as sources of labor and resources and are diversifying their economies. The world economy is rapidly trending toward a multipolar one.[17]

The National Intelligence Council[17] notes a paradox in that some Americans view globalization, immigration, and access to information as trends to be opposed. They prefer polices that they hope will return the world economy to American dominance.[17] Some have turned to nationalism, seeking control over who and what enter the country. Others have embraced populism, supporting policies that address their values and preferences which they feel are not represented. Our seventh point is an assertion that nationalism and populism will likely increase in the foreseeable future.

Unprecedented change is a clear challenge for creating Health in All Policies and building a culture of health. Science and technology will continue to accelerate research, but there is a need to temper the marketing of their findings until objective evaluations are made to be sure they do not harm the health and welfare of the population. Cognitive scientist Paul Smaldino blames the culture of the scientific community for publishing exciting results in prestigious journals before the claims of benefit have been properly vetted.[20] Similarly, products are often rushed to market without careful safety review.[21] The recent case of the Boeing 737 MAX plane illustrates that rushing to market can sometimes have extraordinarily painful consequences.[22] Of course, the pain subsides for the party that increased the risk when the government steps in to provide them with resources.

Those who adamantly support reducing human risk are in a struggle with those who want to hear only about the consequences they value, often economic ones. We need to break this impasse steeped in political tribalism. Although it will not be easy, we need to pursue civil exchanges as the alternative to groupthink, a process that may be counterproductive to improving the health of the population. As an example, consider the case of hydroxychloroquine. The evidence for benefits or harms for the drug's use in COVID-19 patients was very weak and conflicting.[23] However, groupthink pushed many to view the drug as a magic bullet, so they hoarded it, creating a shortage for the patients who needed it to treat systemic lupus erythematosus.[24]

How do we make civil interchanges among the political tribes happen? This remains a conundrum, especially when many people are fixed in their beliefs and many do not vote. Persuading people to vote (in person or by mail) in federal, state, and local elections regardless of party would be a good start. Voting to express our concerns and values is something we should all believe in.

Cascading Environmental Threats

Beginning in the late nineteenth century, government initiated four major eras in U.S. environmental protection. President Theodore Roosevelt acted to set aside natural parks. Decades later, President Franklin Roosevelt addressed serious floods and the Great Depression by developing flood control programs. During the 1970s, President Richard Nixon signed pollution control legislation that addressed multiple air, water, and soil contaminants.[25] Some national, state, and local governments are now fighting the battle of global climate change. This issue, along with that of nuclear weapons, may be the ultimate challenge for humankind. We currently face environmental threats posed by limited freshwater access, toxic waste sites, indoor air pollution, contamination of the lower atmosphere, epidemics and pandemics, pesticides, genetically modified organisms, nanomaterials, and others.

We lack a solid understanding of how these problems cascade. To address this lack of understanding, we need to develop new risk estimates that include multiple hazards at multiple scales for multiple time periods. These estimates need to include levels of uncertainty for various combinations of hazards, times, and places.[26] Unfortunately, most researchers and policymakers focus on a limited number of these challenges—typically climate change or cyber threats. They fail to recognize that a sustainable solution for one problem may exacerbate others. We strongly believe that developing an agenda that considers the breadth of environmental problems and tries to find solutions through public-private partnerships among multiple disciplines and across geographical scales is the right approach to addressing environmental cascades.[27-29] It will be difficult to achieve these partnerships, but without them we will continue to fall into intersecting environmental problems with undeniable health effects.

For example, we lack a solid understanding of the vulnerability of both remote islands and large urban centers in the climate change era. These threatened locales suffer from a decline in marine species; non-native species invasions; destruction of land–ocean interfaces for housing, ports, waste sites, and other uses; population change and migration; and lack of resources, especially fresh water. These pressing issues require answers based on detailed science, forward-thinking planning, and broad public engagement from residents. A Health in All Policies approach for these highly vulnerable places is imperative because it may not be too late for them to take palliative actions.

A U.S. example is the need for multidisciplinary work to understand potentially cascading environmental effects resulting from intensification of dense urban development. Here the issues include the loss of open space, important ecosystems, water resources, and cultural heritage. Smart growth means planning to limit environmental degradation due to sprawl, yet it requires more than inhibiting growth at the edge of the region. Success requires rehabilitating some downtowns, providing transit-oriented development, and increasing the capacity of older city schools. In some places it requires new options for walking and biking, encouraging infill projects, and building interactions among mayors as well as county and state officials to coordinate these activities.

Social scientists must be part of the solution to help officials make better decisions about complex cascading problems because they are the ones who examine economic, social, and political impacts that carry weight with some decision-makers. Coupling science, engineering, and social science talents has already produced effective solutions to reducing air, water, and land emissions by employing pollution-prevention alternatives such as employing recycling and using less resource-intensive and safer production processes. We believe that advocates for Health in All Policies and a culture of health will be at the core of this effort because they tend to use mile-high visioning that includes multidisciplinary experts capable of connecting intersecting issues.

Growing Disparities in Economic, Social, and Political Access

The past sixty years have witnessed marked increases in wealth and educational achievement across the nation, although the distribution is remarkably askew.[30–34] Former Secretary of Labor Robert Reich[34] stated that 95 percent of economic gains went to the top 1 percent in net worth in the decade following the recovery that began in 2009. Extremely affluent Americans continue to widen the wealth gap by using political power to maintain their access to the most prestigious schools, the best opportunities, the homes in desirable neighborhoods, and excellent medical care. They form enclaves that are not geographically located, communicating digitally instead of traveling to a central office and maintaining the flexibility to move in order to minimize their taxes.

The Pew Research Center's 2018 report[32,33] defines middle class as having a family income of two-thirds to double the national median family income ($48,000 to $145,000 in 2018 dollars for a family of three). New Jersey's median family income is higher, but so is the state's cost of living. Over 70 percent of New Jersey families with an income of $100,000 or more have two working family members, often with extended hours to pay the higher taxes, housing, health, auto and other transportation costs, plus the costs of education. A recent OECD study[30] reported that, compared with other countries, middle-income Americans suffer from low-income growth, reduced job security, and rising costs. Nobel Prize economist Angus Eaton[31] created an "unfair" scale with healthcare financing at the top of his unfair list. The middle class is struggling to keep up. Will they be able to keep their jobs, climb an organizational ladder, raise a family, own a home, take an annual vacation, and afford health care? Those not in the top 1 percent justly feel insecure.

If current trends continue it is hard to see how the middle class will not slip downward and how the poor will be able to escape their economic status. Automation threatens repetitive jobs of all types and more Americans with poverty status. Poverty is associated with poor health and a diminished quality of life because the poor often lack access to good schools, housing, health services, and disease-prevention programs. The poor often lack access to fresh food and to opportunities and services.

Socioeconomic status (SES) is the most predictive correlate of health outcomes. Indeed, where you live matters, and there is clear evidence that how long you live may depend on your zip code.[35] Disparities in SES are continuing to increase and are likely to remain a critical influence on health in New Jersey for the foreseeable future. Consider the impact of COVID-19 and its variants on people in the lower income brackets. These individuals are often employed as healthcare workers, grocery store workers, and delivery drivers, placing them at increased risk for exposure to agents of disease. They also work in restaurant, hospitality, retail, and other service industries that have been cut, putting them at risk for a loss of income they cannot afford.[36]

The modern U.S. economy clearly privileges well-educated and highly skilled people, and outcomes are measured in material gains. How Health in All Policies and a culture of health can make a difference, we think, depends on our ability to elect candidates who are aware of and deeply care about the chasm in SES, its impact on future generations, and the nation's overall quality of life and competitiveness. Pressure from an engaged electorate, particularly those with the most to lose, can make an enormous difference in moving policies forward that improve the health of the state.

Demographic Change

Seventy-six million Americans were born between 1946 and 1964, the largest birth cohort in U.S. history. These baby boomers constitute one-fourth of the U.S. population. It is fair to say that their preferences and needs have driven national, state, local, and business priorities, including the proliferation of automobiles, highways, and suburban housing and malls, the development of the Sunbelt, and the decline of older cities. We can, however, credit them with a commitment to environmental protection.

Boomers are declining in numbers, but their legacy continues, especially in regard to their impact on healthcare budgets, their need for downsized affordable housing, and their need to navigate without a personal automobile. Developers in states like New Jersey, New York, California, and others are building condominiums and apartments that can transition to nursing care facilities.[37] Some boomers are former suburbanites who are settling in cities, but many have kept their suburban preferences and are moving to more tax-friendly states or special developments.[38,39] Transportation systems are adapting by offering buses and taxi services to help with mobility. If cities lose their reputation as dangerous places, baby boomers may choose to relocate in cities near shopping, medical, and other services.[40-43]

The second major demographic trend is shrinking household size, from 3.37 in 1950 to 2.63 in 2021.[44] Married couples with children made the biggest decline during that period, replaced by couples without children, single-parent families, and one-person households. Pew Research[44] notes the rise in the number of multigenerational families, particularly from the Great Recession which forced more people into shared living quarters. In 2019, 20 percent of households were shared, often by young adults remaining with their parents. The current configuration of households has been somewhat of a surprise to the construction industry. Dan Parolek, a California architect, notes that developers are fixated on big units and resist changing their business model. Instead, they are missing the untapped market for high-quality, smaller units to serve smaller households.[45] COVID-19 could steer some developers back to smaller units.

The third trend in the United States is diversity, even if immigration is restricted. We cannot say how this diversity will play out, but people with resources will likely settle where they feel most comfortable with regard to SES as well as race/ethnicity/nationality. There are likely to be more multi-cultural identity neighborhoods, such as in Jersey City, for younger people. Yet the suburbs will continue as bastions of political power and wealth, allowing suburbanites to promote their own communities and distance themselves from city problems.

Richard Nixon's power base was the suburbs, and his "new" federalism allocated federal dollars to states where suburban-dominated legislatures could distribute it. In New Jersey, the wealth-belt suburban counties and the southern counties may not be so ready to embrace Health in All Policies or build a culture of health because they perceive these movements as leading to unwarranted transfer payments to cities. For example, the New Jersey Supreme Court stepped up to make the policy decisions that the legislature would not in the cases of Mount Laurel and Abbott. The state government has made it difficult to develop in the Pinelands and the upland watersheds in the Raritan Basin, steps not viewed favorably by many in the wealth-belt and southern counties. Health in All Policies and a culture of health approach can play major roles in focusing legislative attention on the implications of demographic change on health. It requires building a broad political base to show that healthier people will increase the aggregate wealth in the state in the long run.

Politics, Power, and Hedgehog and Fox Strategies

What is the purpose of power in the United States at this time? Depending on the sources consulted, the answers can be remarkably different. Some believe the purpose of power is to serve their self-interest; others believe it is to make as many people as happy as possible.[46] Some act as though the purpose of political power is to grow income, jobs, and other economic assets; others demand attention to social, environmental, and security concerns as well as prosperity. In the United States, we expect disagreement over the goals of power, which dates back to our nation's origin.

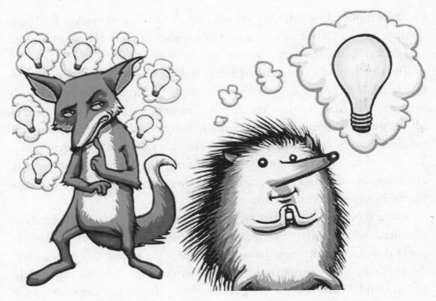

FIGURE E.1 Fox and hedgehog strategic thinking. (*Source:* Pilkington (2016).[50])

Today, we find it hard to discern a grand strategy behind politics in the United States. Isiah Berlin's essay on Tolstoy's view of history distinguished between hedgehogs and foxes.[47] Hedgehogs know one big thing—in the case of politics, it might be some kind of divine plan or totalitarianism—and they use it to organize their thinking and actions. By contrast, foxes know a bit about many things—they are flexible about their choices, and they are open to suggestions and changes (Figure E.1). John Lewis Gaddis[48] similarly classified famous leaders of the past into these two groups: he characterized Abraham Lincoln and Franklin D. Roosevelt as foxes in the face of uncertainty, whereas the twentieth-century totalitarians who ruled the Soviet Union and Germany he labeled hedgehogs. Gaddis praised the authors of the *Federalist Papers* for producing a work of grand strategy because they balanced high aspirations and limited capacities.[49]

Currently, the United States and many state and local governments appear to have many hedgehogs with narrowly directed aspirations and no grand strategy, except to garner more power. Governing the United States is difficult without a single goal to galvanize public attention. Today that focus appears to be on growing the economy, with values on one side embedded in nationalist and populist principles. On the flip side of that focus are values steeped in progressivism. Both sides have strong views about immigration, environmental protection, and social programs.[51] Both take advantage of the digital world, using communication tools to build digital walls around their values and harden their political identities.[52] The loser in this battle of political will is a grand strategy of long-term mutual understanding, greater tolerance and diversity, and collaboration—concepts necessary to support human physical, mental, and social health.

The alternative to narrowly defined agendas is to draw together individuals and build flexible groups to achieve common goals. In this vein, we believe that Health in All Policies and building a culture of health are grand strategies that foxes must use to demonstrate morally and scientifically grounded findings that will attract widespread public support for policies that move us to a healthier New Jersey.

To summarize, the grand strategy for improving the health of all New Jersey residents over the next twenty-five years is to seek out and create opportunities to advance a Health in All Policies agenda and to be prepared to adapt to change as the process unfolds. Although we still have much to learn about the upstream and social determinants of health, we now have the tools to create the policies and culture needed to move us toward a healthier future.

References

1 Osterholm MT. Preparing for the Next Pandemic. *Foreign Affairs*, June 1, 2005. https://www.foreignaffairs.com/articles/2005-07-01/preparing-next-pandemic

2 Osterholm MT, Olshaker M. Chronic of a Pandemic Foretold. *Foreign Affairs*, July/August, 2020. https://www.foreignaffairs.com/search/Chronic of a Pandemic Foretold

3 Sachs JD. Chapter 7. Addiction and unhappiness in America. In: *The World Happiness Report*. Sustainable Development Solutions Network; 2019. https://worldhappiness.report/ed/2019/addiction-and-unhappiness-in-america/

4 Goldman L. *Too Much of a Good Thing: How Four Key Survival Traits Are Now Killing Us*. Boston: Little, Brown; 2015.

5 Alter A. *Irresistible: The Rise of Addictive Technology and the Business of Keeping US Hooked*. New York: Penguin; 2018.

6 Sussman SY. *Substance and Behavioral Addictions: Concepts, Causes, and Cures*. Cambridge: Cambridge University Press; 2017.

7 Institute for Health Metrics and Evaluation. GBD Results Tool. GHDx, 2017. Accessed August 3, 2020. http://ghdx.healthdata.org/gbd-results-tool

8   Babic R, Babic D, Martinac M, et al. Addictions without drugs: contemporary addictions or way or life? *Psychiatr Danub*. 2018;30(Suppl 6):371–379. http://www.psychiatria-danubina.com/UserDocsImages/pdf/dnb_vol30_noSuppl 6/dnb_vol30_noSuppl 6_371.pdf

9   Ennett ST, Tobler NS, Ringwalt CL, Flewelling RL. How effective is drug abuse resistance education? A meta-analysis of Project DARE outcome evaluations. *Am J Public Health*. 1994;84(9):1394–1401. doi:10.2105/ajph.84.9.1394

10 West SL, O'Neal KK. Project D.A.R.E. outcome effectiveness revisited. *Am J Public Health*. 2004;94(6):1027–1029. doi:10.2105/ajph.94.6.1027

11 Fishbein M, Hall-Jamieson K, Zimmer E, et al. Avoiding the boomerang: testing the relative effectiveness of antidrug public service announcements before a national campaign. *Am J Public Health*. 2002;92(2):238–245. doi:10.2105/ajph.92.2.238

12 Matthews S, Dwyer R, Snoek A. Stigma and self-stigma in addiction. *J Bioeth Inq*. 2017;14(2):275–286. doi:10.1007/s11673-017-9784-y

13 Hogg M. Radical change: the search for social identity leads to "Us" versus "Them." *Sci Am*. 2019;321(3):84–87. https://www.scientificamerican.com/article/the-search-for-social-identity-leads-to-us-versus-them/

14 Kose MA, Ozturk EO. A world of change. *Financ Dev*. 2014;51(3):6–11. https://www.imf.org/external/pubs/ft/fandd/2014/09/kose.htm

15 Louv R. *Last Child in the Woods*. New York: Algonquin Press; 2008.

16 Schilhab T. Digital knowledge is a poor substitute for learning in the real world. *Science Nordic*, January 9, 2018. https://sciencenordic.com/denmark-forskerzonen-learning/digital-knowledge-is-a-poor-substitute-for-learning-in-the-real-world/1452971

17 National Intelligence Council. *Global Trends: Paradox of Progress*. NIC 2017-001. Washington, DC: NIC; 2017. https://www.dni.gov/files/documents/nic/GT-Full-Report.pdf

18 Bown CP, Irwin DA. Trump's assault on the global trading system. *Foreign Aff*. 2019;98(5):125–136. https://www.foreignaffairs.com/articles/asia/2019-08-12/trumps-assault-global-trading-system

19 Lagutina ML. BRICS in a world of regions. *Third World Thematics*. 2019;4(6):442–458. doi:10.1080/23802014.2019.1643781

20 Smaldino PE, McElreath R. The natural selection of bad science. *R Soc Open Sci*. 2016;3(9):160384. doi:10.1098/rsos.160384

21 Booty L. Rushed to market product recall disasters: slow and steady wins the race. *Business Advice*, September 29, 2016. https://businessadvice.co.uk/business-development/sales-marketing/rushed-to-market-product-recall-disasters-slow-and-steady-wins-the-race/

22 House Committee on Transportation & Infrastructure. The Boeing 737 MAX Aircraft: Costs, Consequences, and Lessons from Its Design, Development, and Certification. Preliminary Investigative Findings. March 2020. https://transportation.house.gov/imo/media/doc/TI Preliminary Investigative Findings Boeing 737 MAX March 2020.pdf

23 Hernandez AV, Roman YM, Pasupuleti V, et al. Hydroxychloroquine or chloroquine for treatment or prophylaxis of COVID-19: a living systematic review. *Ann Intern Med*. 202018;173(4):287–296. doi:10.7326/M20-2496

24 Peschken CA. Possible consequences of a shortage of hydroxychloroquine for patients with systemic lupus erythematosus amid the COVID-19 pandemic. *J Rheumatol.* 2020;47(6):787–790. doi:10.3899/jrheum.200395

25 Dunlap RE, Mertig AG. The evolution of the U.S. environmental movement from 1970 to 1990: an overview. *Soc Nat Resour.* 1991;4(3):209–218. doi:10.1080/08941929109380755

26 Haimes YY. *Modeling and Managing Interdependent Complex Systems of Systems.* Hoboken, NJ: Wiley/IEEE Press; 2018.

27 Institute of Medicine. *Global Environmental Health in the 21st Century.* Washington, DC: National Academies Press; 2007. doi:10.17226/11833

28 National Academy of Sciences, National Academy of Engineering, and Institute of Medicine. *Preparing for the 21st Century: The Environment and the Human Future.* Washington, DC: National Academies Press; 1997. doi:10.17226/9536

29 Matson P. Environmental challenges for the twenty-first century: interacting challenges and integrative solutions. *Ecol Law Q.* 2001;27:1179–1190. doi:10.2307/24114055

30 OECD. *Under Pressure: The Squeezed Middle Class.* Paris: OCED Publishing; 2019. doi:10.1787/689afed1-en

31 Eaton A. A Nobel Prize-winning economist thinks we're asking all the wrong questions. *Protectors of Equality in Government,* December 28, 2017. https://equalityingov.org/2017/12/a-nobel-prize-winning-economist-thinks-were-asking-all-the-wrong-questions/

32 Matthau D. Are you middle class? Depends where you live in NJ. *New Jersey 101.5,* September 19, 2019. https://nj1015.com/are-you-middle-class-depends-where-you-live-in-nj/

33 Kochhar R. Middle class keeps its size, loses financial ground to upper-income tier. Pew Research Center, September 6, 2018. https://www.pewresearch.org/fact-tank/2018/09/06/the-american-middle-class-is-stable-in-size-but-losing-ground-financially-to-upper-income-families/

34 Reich RB. *The Common Good.* New York: Alfred A. Knopf; 2018.

35 USALEEP: The United States Small-Area Life Expectancy Project. NAPHSIS, 2021. https://www.naphsis.org/usaleep

36 Garfield R, Rae M, Claxton G, Orgera K. Double Jeopardy: Low Wage Workers at Risk for Health and Financial Implications of COVID-19. Kaiser Family Foundation, April 29, 2020. https://www.kff.org/coronavirus-covid-19/issue-brief/double-jeopardy-low-wage-workers-at-risk-for-health-and-financial-implications-of-covid-19/

37 How continuing care retirement communities work. AARP, January 27, 2022. https://www.aarp.org/caregiving/basics/info-2017/continuing-care-retirement-communities.html

38 Horan S. Where retirees are moving. *SmartAsset,* March 10, 2020. https://smartasset.com/financial-advisor/where-retirees-are-moving-2020

39 Jackson C. The suburbs are coming to a city near you. *New York Times,* May 5, 2019. https://www.nytimes.com/2019/05/18/opinion/sunday/the-suburbs-cities.html

40 Sivaramakrishnan K. *As the World Ages: Rethinking a Demographic Crisis.* Cambridge, MA: Harvard University Press; 2018.

41 Lutz W, Sanderson WC, Scherbov S. *The End of World Population Growth in the 21st Century: New Challenges for Human Capital Formation and Sustainable Development.* New York: Routledge/Earthscan; 2004.

42 Lutz W, Goujon A, Samir KC, et al. *Demographic and Human Capital Scenarios for the 21st Century: 2018 Assessment for 201 Countries.* EUR 29113 EN. Luxembourg: Publications Office of the European Union; 2018. doi:10.2760/835878

43 Blossfeld H-P, Buchholz S, Hofäcker D. *Globalization, Uncertainty and Late Careers in Society.* New York: Routledge; 2006.

44 Fry R. U.S. household size is increasing for first time in at least 160 years. Pew Research Center, October 1, 2019. https://www.pewresearch.org/fact-tank/2019/10/01/the-number-of-people-in-the-average-u-s-household-is-going-up-for-the-first-time-in-over-160-years/

45 Sisson P. Why we can't build small homes anymore. *Curbed,* March 10, 2020. https://www.curbed.com/2020/3/10/21168519/homes-for-sale-american-home-suburbs

46 Lindström L. The goal of politics: making people happy. *The Local,* September 26, 2007. https://www.thelocal.se/20070926/8611

47 Berlin I. *The Hedgehog and the Fox: An Essay on Tolstoy's View of History.* London: Weidenfeld & Nicolson; 1953.

48 Gaddis JL. *On Grand Strategy.* New York: Penguin; 2018.

49 Hamilton A, Madison J, Jay J, et al. *The Federalist Papers.* New York: Signet Classics; [1787] 2003.

50 Pilkington G. Accomplishment's secret couriers: "The Hedgehog and the Fox." *Medium,* November 1, 2016. https://medium.com/the-mission/accomplishments-secret-couriers-the-hedgehog-and-the-fox-c7b61a8d8002

51 Xiaonan W. What's in store: globalization, parochialism, or somewhere in between? CGTM, February 23, 2019. https://news.cgtn.com/news/3d3d414f776b444f32457a6333566d54/index.html

52 Clarke RA, Knake R. The internet freedom league: how to push back against the authoritarian assault on the web. *Foreign Aff.* 2019;98(5):184–192. https://www.foreignaffairs.com/print/node/1124537

Acknowledgments

The authors would like to thank two lions in the field of public health for their helpful comments and critical review of this book: Dr. Bernard Goldstein, professor and dean emeritus at the University of Pittsburgh Graduate School of Public Health, and Dr. Thomas A. Burke, professor and associate chair at the Johns Hopkins Bloomberg School of Public Health, Department of Health Policy and Management.

Index

Note: Page numbers followed by *f* and *t* indicate a figure or table on the designated page.

Prevention (CDC): data collection
efforts, 37; funding for Plan4Health
project, 212; leading health indicators,
metrics, 4, 6; monitoring of COVID-19,
115–116, 121, 174–175; role in gathering,
disseminating information, 184; role in
launching Mobilizing for Action
through Planning and Partnerships, 211
Centers for Medicare & Medicaid Services,
204
central business districts (CBDs), 59, 61–62
Cerf, Christopher, 143
Certificate of Need (CON) process, 196
Charity Care Law (1978), 192
Chemical Control incinerator explosion,
91–92
chemical manufacturing: air pollution and,
90; cancer and, 43, 82, 84
children: Abbott Preschool program for,
141–142; benefits of CARES Act for,
126; COVID-19 vaccination data, 121,
123; effects of health disparities on,
123–124, 126; efforts at reducing
educational disparities for, 138; exposure
to toxic levels of lead, 114; impact of
home environments, 152; leading health
indicators, 5t; outpatient facilities for,
208; social influences, 33t; studies of
migrant first-generation children, 87
Children's Health Insurance Program
(CHIP), 191
Christie, Chris, 142–143, 148; attempt at
blocking funding for Abbott School
Districts, 142–143; comment about the
COAH criteria, 148; signing of the
POLST law, 199–200
cigarette smoking, 5t, 17, 32t, 38, 87, 97–98,
152
Clean Air Act (1970), 85
climate change: challenges presented by,
viii, 16, 18, 126–127, 165, 181; COVID-19
and, 184; EPA's report on, 172–173;
global warming and, 46–47; weather,
weather-related events and, 169–173
Clinton, Bill, 198t
COH tool, 90–91
community health improvement plans
(CHIPS), 211–212

community health needs assessments
(CHNAs), 211–212
Comprehensive Environmental Response
Compensation and Liability Act
(CERCLA) (1980), 92
Congress of New Urbanism, 70–71
Coronavirus Aid, Relief, and Economic
Security (CARES) Act (2020), 126
Corzine, John, 68, 99, 147
Council on Affordable Housing (COAH),
147–148
COVID-19 pandemic: death rates, 35–36,
112–113, 117–118, 119t, 121, 204; disease
forecasting model, 122–123; domestic
violence and, 114; effects on children,
123–124, 126; effects on college students,
125; effects on education, 36, 116, 118,
123–124, 127–128; effects on educational
opportunity, 123–124; effects on
employment, 125–126; effects on
housing, 123–124, 127–128; effects on
mental health, 124–125; effects on
poverty, 125; effects on schools, 117,
123–124; effects on the economy, 123, 127,
129f; health disparities in NJ during,
118–120; herd immunity and, 120–123;
impact of, viii, 35–36; New York City
infection rates, 116–117; opioid use and,
114; pre-pandemic health disparities in
NJ, 108–111; race-related odds of dying
from, 117; shift to endemic status, ix;
spread of, in New Jersey, 117–118;
states-level deaths comparison, 116;
testing results/data, 174; vaccines/
vaccination for, 120–123, 125–127,
174–175, 204, 208, 219; WHO recognition of, 118–120
COVID-19 vaccinations: creation of, 175;
herd immunity and, 120; national goal,
121; New Jersey goal (2021), 120; race/
ethnicity comparisons, 121–122; state
comparisons, 120–121
Cronkite, Walter, 191
Cross Bronx Expressway (CBE), 63, 65
culture of health: Cancer Alley concern
and, 89; challenges in building, 18, 224,
229; importance of building, 219–221;
Lavizzo-Mourey's call for building, 15;

need for healthier transportation landscape design, 70–71; needs for improvements, 14; overall ranking, 34–35; water transport, 42. *See also* New Jersey Transit (NJT) system
trauma, comprehensive care centers, 205–206, 207*t*

Uncompensated Care Trust Fund (New Jersey), 192–193
United States (U.S.): addictive behaviors metrics, 221–223; Clean Air Act, 85; COVID-19 health disparities, 115–118; disability-adjusted life years (DALYs) data, 222; Emergency Medical Treatment and Active Labor Act, 193; Environmental Protection Agency, ix, 46, 85, 92, 100, 114, 172–173; Federal-Aid (Interstate) Highway Act, 56, 58–59; Federal Emergency Management Agency, 181, 183–184; Federal Housing Administration program, 59; global healthcare costs comparison, 11–13; health care legislation, 197*t*–199*t*; healthcare sector policy timeline, 192–196; Housing Act, 59, 62; impact of demographic change, 228–229; interstate highway system, 57–59, 70, 84; National Air Sampling Network, 85; National

Cancer Act, 86; Nuclear Regulatory Commission, 164; opinions on the purpose of power in, 229–231; Public Health Services, 3; timeline of health care legislation, 197*t*–199*t*
U.S. News & World Report survey, 8–10
U.S. Public Health Service, 3

vaccines/vaccination: for COVID-19, 120–123, 125–127, 174–175, 204, 208, 219; for DTap, polio, MMR, Hib, HelB, varicella, PCV, 5*t*; herd immunity and, 120; for influenza, 32*t*, 38, 109, 110*t*, 128, 173–175; for measles, 120; for pneumonia, 109, 110*t*, 128
Virginia Commonwealth's Center (VCU) on Society and Health, 149–150

water pollution, 74, 94, 97
weather, weather-related events, 169–173
Whitman, Christine Todd, 46, 82–93, 99, 142
Willingboro Township, New Jersey, 59, 60
World Health Organization (WHO), 2
World Trade Center attack (2001), 44, 165, 168, 175–176

Yale University Program on Climate Change, 46–47

About the Authors

MICHAEL R. GREENBERG is distinguished professor emeritus at the Bloustein School, Rutgers University. He studies environmental health and risk analysis, has written more than thirty-five books and more than 350 journal articles, served as editor-in-chief of *Risk Analysis*, and served as both associate dean and dean of the Bloustein School.

DONA SCHNEIDER is professor emeritus at the Bloustein School, Rutgers University. A medical geographer and epidemiologist, she has written nine books and more than 100 journal articles, performed editorial functions for several journals, and served as both associate dean at the Bloustein School and dean of the University College Community.